Promoting Resilience
in Dementia Care

of related interest

Communication Skills for Effective Dementia Care
A Practical Guide to Communication and Interaction Training (CAIT)
Edited by Ian Andrew James and Laura Gibbons
ISBN 978 1 78592 623 5
eISBN 978 1 78592 624 2

CLEAR Dementia Care©
A Model to Assess and Address Unmet Needs
Dr Frances Duffy
ISBN 978 1 78592 276 3
eISBN 978 1 78450 576 9

Sharing Sensory Stories and Conversations with People with Dementia
A Practical Guide
Joanna Grace
ISBN 978 1 78592 409 5
eISBN 978 1 78450 769 5

Teaching Empathy and Conflict Resolution to People with Dementia
A Guide for Person-Centered Practice
Cameron Camp and Linda Camp
ISBN 978 1 78592 788 1
eISBN 978 1 78450 737 4

Enhancing Health and Wellbeing in Dementia
A Person-Centred Integrated Care Approach
Dr Shibley Rahman
Forewords by Professor Sube Banerjee and Lisa Rodrigues
Afterword by Lucy Frost
ISBN 978 1 78592 037 0
eISBN 978 1 78450 291 1

Positive Psychology Approaches to Dementia
Edited by Chris Clarke and Emma Wolverson
Foreword by Christine Bryden
ISBN 978 1 84905 610 6
eISBN 978 1 78450 077 1

Promoting Resilience

— IN —

Dementia Care

A Person-Centred Framework for Assessment and Support Planning

JULIE CHRISTIE

Forewords by Wendy Mitchell and Mary Marshall

Jessica Kingsley Publishers
London and Philadelphia

First published in 2020
by Jessica Kingsley Publishers
73 Collier Street
London N1 9BE, UK
and
400 Market Street, Suite 400
Philadelphia, PA 19106, USA

www.jkp.com

Library of Congress Cataloging in Publication Data
A CIP catalog record for this book is available from the Library of Congress

British Library Cataloguing in Publication Data
A CIP catalogue record for this book is available from the British Library

ISBN 978 1 78592 600 6
eISBN 978 1 78592 601 3

Printed and bound in Great Britain

In memory of my grandparents Margaret and William Wilson, and Anne and James Christie. And to the present day, for Ewan and Finn Stevenson, a couple of great nephews.

Contents

Foreword by Wendy Mitchell 9

Foreword by Professor Mary Marshall 11

Acknowledgements 13

Preface 15

The Resilience Model 19

Introduction: What is Resilience? 23

1. A Brief History of Resilience 31

2. Re-Imagining Resilience: New Concepts and Connections 45

3. The Experience of Threat and Dementia 61

4. Holding on to a Sense of Self 73

5. Protective Factors in Action 83

6. Locating Resilience in Everyday Stories 105

7. Practice Tensions in the Search for Resilience 127

8. Realising Resilience: Practice Scenarios 143

9. The Road to Resilience: Where to from Here? 159

Glossary 169

Bibliography 173

Subject Index 183

Author Index 190

Foreword

When people hear the word 'dementia' they frequently think of the losses, the lack of ability, deterioration. What doesn't come to mind immediately is the ability to adapt, to fight the condition through resilience. When I was diagnosed, I too believed it to be the end, because no one told me any different. However, I soon realised that I wasn't prepared to give into this cruel disease and instead see it now as a game: a game of trying to outwit and outmanoeuvre dementia. When a problem arises, that others may see as a loss, I find a solution, an alternative way. I'm often saying, 'There's always a way', and this applies to many challenges people face in life, but especially dementia. Many people are naturally resilient and creative and those who aren't naturally need support to believe there's alternatives to just giving up. So where should positivity begin? Well, as in most circumstances, the beginning. The person receiving a diagnosis needs hope, not despair, which is sadly usually the case as healthcare professionals offer little in the way of positivity when delivering a diagnosis.

This book is refreshingly powerful in positivity; positivity shines through, showing how, through support and understanding, we can 'live' and not just 'exist' with dementia. The small change of one word that could help someone see that a diagnosis of dementia is, yes, a hard diagnosis to receive, but can also be the start of a different way of living. We can be given the support and strength to see how resilience, our resilience, that has seen us through many trials in our life previously, can now be used to live with dementia.

Wendy Mitchell
Author of *Sunday Times* best-seller *Somebody I Used to Know*

Foreword

In 1982 I took a sabbatical from teaching social work and worked in Victoria in Australia, attached to the social work department of an old age psychiatry hospital. I lived in a housekeeper's flat: pleasant but wholly impersonal. It was great to have six months being a different person since I knew nobody before I went. I still, however, recall returning home and being back again amongst my possessions. I felt an overwhelming sense of relief at being reminded of who I really was. I was therefore enchanted by Julie Christie's mention of objects as part of resilience assessment.

The Australia trip was life changing for other reasons. I discovered alternative models of care which were based on people's competence rather than incompetence. There were family group homes where people shared chores as far as they could, there were housing models and community day facilities. All very different from the UK at the time where almost all care was in hospitals and the focus was almost exclusively on supporting carers since there was a very pessimistic view taken of dementia. I returned determined to promote this more social model where the focus of assessment was much wider than what was going on in the brain. Life skills, background history, relationships, personality and so on are seen as crucially part of the experience of dementia. This approach is now mainstream but there is still a tendency to talk about: 'dementia is…' And then to go on about damage to the brain caused by dementia and what are seen as pretty much inevitable symptoms such as loss of memory, reasoning, language skills, etc. In over 30 years of teaching, I have been guilty of these generalisations too.

What is so profoundly encouraging about this book is the emphasis on very careful listening in order to really understand the coping skills of each individual with dementia. Referring to a wide range of research studies and illustrating the necessary skills using lots of stories, Julie Christie shows how we need to listen without assumptions if we are to find the often small and subtle ways we can help people to continue the lives they want to lead. It is the step beyond rehabilitation which has itself had too little traction in dementia care. She embraces, within resilience assessment, a very wide range of factors which can help: in personal strengths, in terms of relationships and in the tangible furniture of all our lives: buildings, objects, food, etc. Yes it takes time, longer than ticking boxes of impairments and needs, but it can also save money and certainly help us caring professionals provide a better service. We need to really believe the phrase we often use about 'everyone's journey through dementia is unique' and to understand that this can be in very subtle ways that need a careful assessment of resilience followed by imaginative and sensitive interventions, if the journey is to be a better one.

Professor Mary Marshall
Author of *Perspectives on Rehabilitation and Dementia*

Acknowledgements

Thank you to my family, Margaret and Ranald Christie, Anne Stevenson and, in particular, my husband Ronnie Stevenson for supporting my passion to bring this book to life.

I want to thank all of the people who gave their time, stories and accounts in the creation of this work. Thank you to my PhD supervisors Dr Brenda Gillies, Dr Fiona Kelly and Professor Brigid Daniel. In particular, the work of Brigid Daniel and Sally Wassell in bringing resilience to life for practitioners working with children and families has been a great inspiration to me in planning and writing this book. Thank you to Dr Richard Ward for his encouragement in finding a publisher and to Tony Keogh for supporting my early research interests.

This research would not have been possible without the contributions of the many people with dementia, the practitioners and academics who found time to meet with me and participate in this process. In particular, Wendy Mitchell and Professor Mary Marshall who have both taken the time to read drafts and write forewords.

Preface

This book is about the resilience of the person living with dementia. What do I mean by this? It's about life with dementia, and the ways in which people who are living with dementia experience adversity and find new ways of coping. It is designed with the full spectrum of health, social work, social care, housing and human service practitioners in mind. It is also set within the context of political, financial and societal reality. Resilience is not a mystical power that renders us invulnerable. Neither does it resolve structural issues that disempower or result in discrimination. Dementia is a progressive condition for which there is currently no cure. People living with dementia and carers require advice, support and access to high-quality care delivered by skilled practitioners. However, people also need to live their life with dementia. This book will explore how this life is experienced through the lens of resilience.

This book has been many years in the making. I have worked with older people and people with dementia for most of my professional life. I qualified as a Mental Health Nurse in 1992 and, after spending some time in the care home sector, moved to a local authority employer to follow my interest in working with people who were living with dementia. At the time this was seen as unusual as dementia wasn't talked about as a career choice. In 1996, I became one of the first nurse care managers in Scotland as hospitals for adults with mental health needs and learning disabilities closed through community care reforms, implemented through the NHS and Community Care Act (1990). I worked as part of a social work team assessing the needs of older people. This was at the height of the new managerialism of social work, where there was an emphasis on the person in receipt of services being re-framed as a consumer (Jacobs *et al.*, 2009), although I was unaware of the politics at the time. I found a home in social work and spent many years as a social worker and a manager of social work teams for older people and hospital social work services. I have worked with people who have just received a diagnosis of dementia, people who have high support needs, people in need of protection and people with dementia at the end of life. This close working with people at intimate moments of their life has been both humbling and rewarding and has taught me much about simply being human.

At the same time, I was also fortunate enough to be able to pursue academic interests. I completed an MSc in Dementia Studies, the first example of such a degree in the world, in 2002. Following this, I worked closely with the Dementia Services Development Centre at the University of Stirling as a teaching assistant, trainer and consultant. I also enjoyed a period of secondment at the centre to develop resources for acute care staff in the care of people with dementia in hospitals. I completed my social work degree in 2005, and during this time I focused on work with children and young adults. It was here that I discovered the work of Daniel and Wassell (2002a, 2002b, 2002c) on resilience. At the time I was struck by what a valuable resource these resilience practice guides were. I used resilience frameworks within my assessments, and court reports, and found the concept both challenging and stimulating. After this introduction to resilience I was keen to discuss with colleagues, in practice and academia, similar frameworks for practice with people with dementia. This quickly led to the realisation that there were no such frameworks. Further, there was some doubt expressed that resilience applied to dementia, and so my PhD journey began. The content of this book is the result of that research, which asked the question, 'Is the concept of resilience applicable to people with dementia?'

A range of political, social and cultural influences brought me to the topic of resilience. It has developed from my interests in citizenship, dementia and practice. Working with people with dementia has enabled me to reflect on the nature of human services work, in particular to ask: are there missed practice opportunities to work in more creative ways with people living with dementia? My own experiences of people who are living with dementia have included reflections on the possibility of resilience and what resilience might mean in the context of living with dementia. Through resilience, we can reveal new insights about life with dementia and, in turn, offer an alternative discourse on both dementia, and the nature of resilience itself. The everyday stories told by people with dementia are potentially unheard demonstrations of resilience in action. These stories are an untapped resource for carers and practitioners who work in the dementia field. I hope that this book provides you with the tools to realise resilience in your practice. Most of all, I hope that this book enables us to create better stories of life with dementia together.

The Resilience Model

In Brief

Resilience is the process of adaptation in the face of adversity. It involves the interaction of a range of risk and protective factors. We can facilitate resilience by reducing risks, and promoting protective factors through targeted resources. We gather these resources throughout our lives. This accumulation of resources can be thought of as our personal Resilience Reserve. We, therefore, all have resources to draw on and the potential for resilience.

In the context of dementia, resilience can be thought of as the process of *adaptation to hold on to a sense of self in the face of threats to identity.*

In order to realise resilience we can:

1. Use the Resilience Reserve to visualise each person's resources (please see Figure 2.1 in Chapter 2).

2. Appraise risk and protective factors and identify areas for attention (please see Table 5.1 in Chapter 5).

3. Use the Resilience Reserve to identify resources that could be employed to reduce risks and promote protective factors.

4. Provide resources that the person needs but does not have.

The Resilience Reserve

Our Resilience Reserve is a personal repository that each of us has to meet the demands and challenges of life. We build this reserve through our knowledge, skills, experiences, networks, assets and resources. The more that we refer to our personal reserve, in order to meet these challenges successfully, the more trust we build that we can meet future challenges.

The Risk and Protective Factors Quick Rating Tool (Table 5.1 in Chapter 5) provides an at-a-glance overview of the risk and protective factors of an individual. Protective factors act as buffers in the face of adversity. The more protective factors that a person has, the more resilient he or she is likely to be. Conversely, risk factors may increase the impact of adversity, causing emotional distress and anxiety, and making it difficult for the person to respond and adapt. With regard to dementia, protective factors fall under three main headings:

- *sense of connectedness* with others

- *sense of mastery and control* over situations and events

- *meaning making* opportunities.

Connectedness is achieved through personal relationships with the people, places and things in our life. This must be rewarding and contribute to our sense of wellbeing. If identity is shaped and reinforced through relationships, then connectedness has an important role with regard to our sense of self. Connectedness includes feeling part of a family, or group or community, knowing that there is someone out there who is thinking of you, or is there for you to fall back on, and importantly, that someone would miss you if you weren't there.

Mastery and control refers to a person's sense of competence and efficacy in a situation: the feeling that in any situation you know what to do, are able to take action, and that that action will result in a change, or have an impact. This also includes how we are able to influence within our network, and being able to mobilise assets, and harness knowledge and skills, to achieve maximum impact.

Meaning making refers to the way in which we make sense of our experiences and interactions with others.

Introduction

What is Resilience?

'Don't get all worried and stressed and think "what if I wake up tomorrow and I can't do that, what if somebody laughs at me" endless worries really but you don't need to go there.'

'Resilience' is a word used often in the context of modern life but what exactly is it? If you were to ask different people you would struggle to find a single definition. Resilience is a vague concept with contradictory explanations. It is little surprise that in our work with people in situations of care and support, it can be hard to use a concept like resilience with confidence. Simply put, resilience can be described as 'bounce back ability': positive adaptation in the face of challenge and adversity (see Luthar *et al.*, 2000). Importantly, resilience is an ordinary phenomenon (Masten, 2001) and as such the concept is applicable to all. So, what might this mean in the context of life with dementia? How can resilience be recognised and harnessed by people with dementia, carers and practitioners? This is what we will explore together in this book. Resilience can be thought of as the process of adaptation to promote wellbeing. We do this through responding and adapting to the stresses and challenges which impact on us and our lives. The important points to remember as we begin are that resilience is:

- an ordinary phenomenon

- a process and not a characteristic

- developed through the experience of adversity in our lives.

Dementia

Dementia results in a range of signs and symptoms, the most common of which is short-term memory loss. People can also experience difficulties with planning, organising and problem solving. Sensory changes can mean that we become more sensitive to the impact of the built and the social environment. Every person is different and experiences different signs and symptoms and to varying degrees, but what everyone shares is the innate human impact of the condition. Lives and relationships are changed, roles, friends and networks can be diminished, but the person and their unique place in the world remains. There are many conditions which cause dementia, and diagnosis can be a complex process, with little reference to a person's existing skills and life experiences, both past and present. People with dementia can be described as 'sufferers' or as a 'burden' to those who care for them, and to wider society in practical and economic terms. People with dementia are not, however, victims of disease or suffering, instead each person is a member of society, or citizen, with the capacity and potential for resilience. The human impact of dementia is, therefore, as important as the clinical description.

Resilience Doesn't Apply to People with Dementia, Does It?

Resilience in the context of dementia is a relatively new field. In the past, when I searched libraries and databases on the subject I was unable to find any resources, and yet there was a wealth of information on the subject of resilience and other groups, especially children. When I asked specifically for dementia and resilience resources, I was advised that they didn't exist as 'resilience didn't apply to people with dementia'. This response certainly did not fit with my own experiences of working with people with dementia and their families, where I could describe people I had known as demonstrating resilience. By this I mean that some people appeared to be living 'a good life' by their own standards, despite dementia. Of course, other people did not. If resilience is an ordinary phenomenon and applicable to all of us, surely there is the possibility of resilience for people living with dementia?

The word 'resilience' can be used when we mean hardiness or invulnerability. Dementia, by comparison, is associated with physical and mental decline, and vulnerability. Resilience is also, wrongly, conflated with the concept of independence, and where this happens, the image of the *dependent person with dementia* is incongruent with this ideal. Externally imposed views of what 'living well' with dementia means, can be unrealistic and, at worst, harmful, for example, a much reduced vision of a good life to a *good enough life* which places an over-emphasis on risk. This can lead to paternalistic approaches and predictable care pathways. A focus is, therefore, required on *this person, living this life* if we are to understand the role that resilience can play. Listening to the experiences and stories of people with dementia can reveal the resilience process and can help us interpret the reasons behind the actions of people with dementia. We can map risk and protective factors for each individual and provide support that builds on strengths, preserves assets and compensates for areas of vulnerability. This book will provide you with the tools to do this.

The Problem with Resilience

'Resilience' must be used with care. Presently, the term is often used incorrectly, because we are unclear about what it means, or use it interchangeably with similar concepts such as recovery, or to signify independence. Resilience can also be used as a value judgement where people are measured against public demonstrations of will power in the face of life adversities. Expectations that people will 'fight the condition' and 'bravely' refuse to give in (or give up). The need for people to be resilient can also be used to compensate for a lack of challenge to inequalities in society or organisational limits on resources. Addressing ageism and the stigma of dementia can then get lost as the 'resilient' person with dementia is expected to cope with attitudes and policies that limit their opportunities.

There is only a very small literature dealing with the subject of resilience in the lives of people with dementia. Instead, we focus on risk, and assessing what people with dementia are no longer able to do. Assessments are used to make a case for the need for resource rather than the need for support. Resilience is also a complex process which requires knowledge of the person and their individual situation. It is context specific, not a fixed state. It includes the interaction of vulnerability and protective factors, and can be promoted and inhibited through the quality of our interactions, care and support. We, therefore, need to understand our own role in facilitating good relationships and fostering an environment for resilience to emerge.

26

Resilience as an Opportunity

Despite the distress and adversity faced by many with dementia, the possibility of resilience remains. Resilience allows us to think differently about the experience of dementia, disrupting the trend to 'hopelessness' that is often heard in the current discourse. At the same time, it also highlights the important role that all of us who work with people with dementia have to play. However, unless this possibility of resilience is acknowledged, and we are equipped with the knowledge and tools to *recognise* resilience, it might never be realised. At its heart, this work brings a focus on the interconnected nature of our lives, as we create opportunities for resilience in relationships with each other. I employ an eco-psycho-social approach to dementia (Zeisel *et al.*, 2016). Dementia, and resilience within the context of dementia, cannot be limited to one domain of human experience. It is contextual, and as such, has to be explored from multiple and overlapping areas of a person's life. It is concerned with citizenship, and the human rights of people with dementia, and recognises the contributions that people with dementia make to their own lives, and to those of other people (see Bartlett and O'Connor, 2007).

Human rights are the basic rights and freedoms that belong to every person in the world, from birth until death. They apply regardless of where you are from, what you believe or how you choose to live your life. These rights are based on our shared values of dignity, fairness, equality, respect and independence and are defined and protected by law. Resilience can help us to recognise and uphold the human rights of people living with dementia. Dementia does not erode our essential personhood, our humanness or our life experiences. Our citizenship also takes many forms, political, social and domestic, as we live our lives, bringing a sharp focus on the experiences of people with dementia in personal spaces, such as the family home. Each of us, even with dementia, has a rich repository of relationships, experiences and knowledge to share. If we ignore this we are missing valuable resources and opportunities to support people to live their life with dementia.

At some time in our lives we will all need to depend on others and the right to care and support is an important part of our society. Resilience-focused practice can also help us to provide timely, targeted support. This occurs when we support strengths, knowledge and skills but also helps us to see and quantify aspects of risks and vulnerabilities in the lives of people with dementia. Resilience is about finding balance and as such is an important tool for practitioners in providing targeted, meaningful and timely support that fits into the lives of people with dementia and carers. Although this book is focused on the person with dementia, the support and wellbeing of carers is also vitally important. You can use the tools in this book to work with carers too and carers can use the tools in building different relationships with the person with dementia that they care for. However, the lack of accessible resilience content for people with dementia directly has been the inspiration for this work.

How to Use This Book

And so, this book is intended to inform the reader on the subject of resilience. An overview of the concept, its origins and the current policy context, is provided in Chapter 1. Chapter 2 explores new concepts in dementia care and practice, their connections and influence on our understanding of resilience. One of these is the concept of the Resilience Reserve, our unique repository of assets and resources. In order to understand resilience, we must first understand the experience of threat and adversity in both ageing and dementia, and so, in Chapter 3, we focus on stories told by people who are living with dementia. Then, in Chapter 4, this discussion expands, re-framing the experience of dementia as a continual process of holding on to a sense of self. The interaction of all of the aforementioned is explained in the 'Dementia Resilience Matrix', a visual framework to understand the elements of a resilience model for dementia.

The second part of this book focuses on resilience in action. In Chapter 5, we explore the protective factors that lessen the impact of threats from the perspective of people living with dementia. This includes the 'Risk and Protective Factors Quick Rating Tool'. This tool enables practitioners to see at a glance areas where a person may have strengths or vulnerabilities, to act on this information, and to communicate this to others. Chapter 6 then explores the ways in which practitioners can discover important information about the person, and the role of assessment in capturing meaningful content to inform resilience. The practical application of resilience in work with people who have dementia is also explored. There are difficulties and challenges in using resilience in practice and we explore these in Chapter 7. Chapter 8 includes practice scenarios to illustrate the ways in which this approach can provide new opportunities to connect both with people with dementia and with carers. Finally, the concluding chapter is an opportunity to reflect on the concept of resilience and its relationship to dementia as we contemplate *where to from here?*

There is a glossary of terms at the end of the book which provides a useful guide for resilience-focused discussions.

In order to illustrate specific points, the voices of people with dementia and care practitioners are used. These examples have been drawn from both my research and practice. Names have been changed and extracts have been used with permission.

CHAPTER 1

A Brief History of Resilience

The word 'resilience' derives from the present participle of the Latin verb *resilire*, meaning to jump back or to recoil. Researchers interested in the psychological and social determinants of health studied the children of parents with schizophrenia. Researchers established the concept of childhood resilience (see, for example, Garmezy, 1974 and Masten *et al.*, 1990) where some children demonstrated better than expected outcomes. By this, the researchers meant that the children did well at school, or had a good network of friends, or appeared to have a good sense of wellbeing, despite their home circumstances. The explanation for this was resilience. As a result, interest grew in the factors at play. What were the specific ingredients that contributed to normal development under adverse circumstances? This data collectively formed the body of knowledge known as 'resilience'. Gradually, researchers turned their attention to the resilience of adults. Early work in this area was concerned with individual characteristics, and discussed resilience as a personal, intrinsic, attribute. There is now a much broader focus, either on factors external to the person that influence resilience, and/or the ways in which we interact with our built and social environments. This includes people, places and things, and our relationship with, and connection to them, informed by cultural and political influences. Resilience is, therefore, a complex interaction of things, constantly evolving as our circumstances change.

The Policy Context

The World Report on Ageing and Health, published by the World Health Organization (WHO) (2015a), highlighted the now important role of resilience in policy conversations on ageing. This is also referred to as healthy ageing. Healthy ageing is defined as 'the process of developing and maintaining the functional ability that enables well-being in older age. Functional ability comprises the health related attributes that enable people to be and to do what they have reason to value' (p.28).

Building resilience is identified in health policies as an essential part of avoiding health problems, in overcoming or bouncing back from inequalities that lead to poor health outcomes, and for living well with frailty as we age (World Health Organization, 2017). The Healthy Ageing model conceptualises resilience as the ability to maintain or improve a level of *functional ability* in the face of adversity, either through a change in attitude, or the ability to call on external resources to compensate for a loss of function. After a fall you might take action within the home to make it safer, such as installing a handrail or thinking differently, for example, 'When I come down the stairs I'm going to be more careful and take things slowly.' Someone else might avoid using the stairs or someone else might consider the accident as a one-off. All of the people here could be described as 'coping' with this scenario, but one person uses their skills, knowledge and contacts to adapt the environment or their behaviour, or both, whilst others cope by avoiding or ignoring the situation.

Older people can also lose their identity when they enter health and care systems. Describing people as 'frail' is a common example. Rahman (2018) raises the stigma of being referred to as 'frail' and the ways in which this might impact on a person's identity. This can also affect how the person is viewed by practitioners. Resilience can be needed to adapt to changes in functional ability, but also to retain a sense of self in the face of attitudes towards older people. Labelling a person as *frail* might be enough to have a negative impact on their self-image, and mean that he or she loses confidence in their own abilities. It is also important to remember that interest in resilience and ageing has grown alongside western, neoliberal health and welfare policies of the late twentieth century, where society views the individual as being responsible for living a healthy lifestyle, in essence, to avoid becoming *frail*, although we all know people who experience ill-health, and require hospital and social care services, despite a healthy lifestyle. As responsible citizens we are expected to accumulate resources over time to ensure our safety and security, and to prevent health problems in the future. When we do experience problems or periods of crisis we can, however, refer to support services and organisations. Our access to these services is now increasingly dependent on demonstrating our eligibility for such support.

We can retain some sense of autonomy when we receive support through initiatives, such as consumer-directed care, or self-directed support. This is where a person receives money from the state to independently make their own care arrangements. As a result, principles of personal accountability (of which resilience could be seen as an example) in matters of social care, health, ageing and disability dominate policy and practice. It is argued that this is an ideological position where the state's role in our private lives (and in the provision of resources) can be minimised, and instead, the resources of each individual are prioritised. Chandler and Reid refer to this as re-defining individuals, not as citizens, but as 'neoliberal subjects' (2016, p.11). Being labelled as *vulnerable* (as opposed to being resilient) can then be thought of as being a person who is unable to overcome personal financial, material or ideological obstacles (p.15) to living an independent life. Independence and resilience appear to be closely linked. This has important implications for life with dementia, and the decisions we make about people with dementia, which we will explore later.

Dementia and Policy

Dementia is a global health priority. At this time there are 27 countries with national dementia plans with many others working on this (Alzheimer Disease International, 2018). There is a focus on dementia prevention through healthy lifestyles, staying connected to communities, main-taining interests and hobbies, staying mentally active (see, for example, Your Brain Matters, a campaign by Dementia Australia: https://yourbrainmatters.org.au); and where dementia is a concern, being able to access a timely diagnosis. When you have dementia, diagnosis is both a fundamental right and an essential entry point to receiving the right advice, care, support and treatment. This includes making legal, practical and financial decisions, as well as recording your preferences for future care and lifestyle choices.

There is much debate about the phrase 'living well' with dementia and its use in a policy context. Resilience is an important aspect of living well, but it doesn't shield you from pain, upset, and the stresses and strains of life. And, of course, not everyone is resilient, and if we understand this, it means that we can appreciate that not everyone can experience wellbeing as they live with dementia. There is also a concern that *living well*, as an aspiration, can place undue pressure on individuals. For some it can feel like an expectation. This can mean that some people don't, or feel that they are not encouraged to, speak openly about feelings of not coping, or grief at the loss of a previous lifestyle. Some might even feel shame, at having *let yourself get dementia*, with all the connotations of old age and senility. Resilience is sometimes used interchangeably with terms such as 'successful ageing' (Havighurst, 1961; Rowe and Khan, 1997), 'active ageing' (Walker, 2006) or 'productive ageing' (Butler, 1969). Older people who then experience ill-health might be considered as having aged unsuccessfully or unproductively. Socio-psychological models of successful ageing focus less on biological processes and disability and more on general life satisfaction, participation and functioning (Bowling and Dieppe, 2005). The indicators applied to determine successful ageing have been debated widely, and could be argued to promote ageist attitudes (Hicks and Conner, 2014). For example, independence and good levels of cognitive functioning are considered as indicators of successful ageing (Bowling and Dieppe, 2005). This can place an unrealistic responsibility on the older person and conditions, such as dementia, might then be seen as a failing on the part of the person concerned (Bavidge, 2006). Resilience is not measured by the absence of ill-health or adversities; instead, it is concerned with the ways in which people achieve better than expected outcomes despite these challenges.

Some people can experience a better quality of life with dementia if we recognise the potential for resilience and support the realisation of resilience. Carers can unintentionally misinterpret the resilient responses of the person concerned, and label changes in behaviour as 'symptoms' of dementia. For example, consider the older woman with dementia who continues to leave her hospital bed, much to the upset of the ward staff and fellow patients. She might be described as 'wandering' or 'disorientated' as a result of dementia. Psycho-social practitioners might consider her restless behaviour as communicating her upset or anxiety. However, a resilience discourse offers another possible answer. The act of moving oneself, and displaying dissatisfaction, can be re-framed as an exercise of power and a strength that can be built into the care planning process. The impact of failing to recognise resilience and only seeing symptoms and responsive behaviours is a cycle of dependence.

The very existence of dementia can mean the potential for resilience is never considered. Most healthcare policies place an emphasis on attending to the physical, mental, social and emotional needs of the person; however, there is not usually an emphasis on resilience, and often no clear definitions or practical guides for people with an interest in this field. Is it possible for resilience to emerge and for practice to mobilise the strengths of the person and their network? Yes, I argue it is, but not without the right tools for the job. In order to help us understand this in more detail we need to look more closely at the impact of ageing.

Resilience, Ageing and Dementia
Attitudes to Ageing

Ellen lives on her own in the same street as her daughter. Her husband Tom died 20 years ago. He had retired from work early due to Parkinson's disease and Ellen cared for him. Ellen's mother lived with the family too and Ellen had cared for both her mum and Tom for a period of time, whilst also raising her son and daughter. Now living on her own, Ellen is enjoying this period of her life, free from responsibilities and able to plan her day to suit herself. She keeps up to date with current affairs as she feels this is important and socialises with friends and neighbours. Recently some of Ellen's friends have experienced ill-health, and last year Ellen received a diagnosis of dementia.

'If people are having a conversation the last thing I would want to do is say, "Oh, I am getting old." No, I'm fairly up to date with what's going on, and as I say I get the paper every morning, watch the television. I think I'm fairly... So really I'm all right. I vary; sometimes I'm quite nice and quite happy but my friends, well, one of them died last year, and the other one, well she's right at the end but she drives and so on. And my neighbours on either side are great. I mean I'm not sitting on their doorstep. I'm quite happy with my own company but I still like to have a chat and a cup of tea.'

Ellen is 81 years old and yet she doesn't want anyone to think she is getting old. Why is this? Society associates ageing with frailty, dependence and ill-health. However, because older people are also members of society they too can be influenced by these stereotypes, and may personally experience ageing accordingly. Butler defined ageism as 'a personal revulsion' to the biological and social consequences of ageing (1969, p.243). The culture of ageism can be described as pervasive and can challenge an individual's sense of self. Sinnot (2009) refers to ageing as a period of uncertainty, and says that, as such, anxiety and anticipatory mourning can be experienced as we grow older. We are also extremely conscious of any cognitive changes in old age. Although some changes can occur, any sign of shortened attention spans, decreased capacity to solve problems, and forgetfulness can promote ageist prejudices, as 'we too readily assume that the differences in attitudes and competencies that characterise old age are deterioration' (Bavidge, 2006, p.48). Again, these prejudices can also be held by older people about themselves, with any changes assumed to be detrimental, threatening the picture that we have of ourselves (Cuddy *et al.*, 2005).

Ageing is not the same for everyone. Neither is ageing made up of either wholly positive or wholly negative experiences. This is also true for those ageing with dementia. Ageing can contribute to strength in the *development* of resilience. This was explored by Bowes and Daniel (2010) and Clark *et al.* (2011). These authors referred to a dimension of resilience which is only understood by thinking about who we are over the course of time. The personal, reflective stories that we share help us to understand ourselves, and help us to predict how we will react in different scenarios. Studies of resilience in old age have focused on bereavement (Bennett, 2010) and adjustments to ill-health and disability (Abbema *et al.*, 2015). More recently research has emerged that addresses adjustments to ageing itself (Windle, 2015). Sources of stress identified include health issues, frailty, retirement, fear of the future, and lack of resources.

Resilience and the Experience of Dementia

Research into resilience and dementia is a relatively new field. The literature on resilience in this area typically discussed the resilience of carers (see, for example, Dias *et al.*, 2015). There is a body of literature on coping with and adjusting to dementia. This work does not explicitly use the term 'resilience', although it does refer to coping with the symptoms of cognitive impairment, and striving to stay the same despite cognitive changes. For example, Pearce *et al.* (2002) discussed the balance between the person with dementia's desire to remain unchanged, and at the same time, their need to re-appraise their view of the world if he or she is to cope with life with dementia. The work of Clare (2003) and Clare and Shakespeare (2004) explained that people with dementia come to terms with their diagnosis and their life with dementia through distinct stages of 'self-maintenance', where the person strives to keep life as before, and, 'adjustment', where the person acknowledges that life cannot continue as before and makes changes. Similarly, Keady *et al.* (2007) explain coping with dementia as an 'act of keeping balance' between the old life and the new, making changes where necessary, but holding on where possible to previous lifestyles. So, the ways in which individuals respond to having dementia depend on their own personal understanding of the situation.

Harris (2008) explored the role of resilience in two case studies of people living with early-stage dementia. She defined resilience as self-reports of 'doing okay' (p.49) and identified dementia as being an adverse event in people's lives. Through a series of open-ended questions, Harris identified vulnerability and protective factors in the lives of each of these two participants, which she considered promoted their continued sense that they were 'doing okay'. She found that both had a positive attitude to having dementia, that they were good at problem solving and had what she described as 'coping skills'. Each person had a positive view of self, they used community resources, and both had positive long-term relationships with their families. Harris hoped that moving to a resilience discourse would change social perceptions of dementia. Yet, despite this, the literature attempting to understand resilience in dementia remains relatively rare. There remains a focus on those in the earlier stages of dementia and resilience in the face of diagnosis. There is still a narrow focus on the individual and their attributes, rather than consideration of dementia as a social experience, where external factors, connections and relationships also shape our Resilience Reserve. One study which did focus on the environment and its role in resilience was that of Clarke and Bailey (2016). This research explored the everyday experiences of living with dementia in rural and semi-urban communities. In summary, this paper highlighted the ways in which places we know well can be both threatening and supportive, as each person with dementia, and their family, negotiate changing roles, relationships and lifestyles.

Where people with dementia contribute to public or academic life as 'a person with dementia', they can be subject to scrutiny and doubt. For example, 'does this person have dementia?' as they don't seem to fit the expectations that we hold about what a person with dementia should be able to do. So, when a person demonstrates resilience, he or she can then find the 'diagnosis' of dementia questioned by others. However, can we re-frame the question and ask if being valued and included can promote resilience? If yes, then *supporting resilience can create resilience*. This is the wonderful opportunity that this untapped area of practice could hold. Resilience can also be in evidence quietly in the struggles of those with a more progressed dementia or at the end of life. Dependence is not an indicator of being more or less resilient, and equally, resilience does not equate to activism or political demonstrations of citizenship. That is why reference to human rights is important.

Dementia, Resilience and Human Rights

According to the Equality and Human Rights Commission, human rights are the basic rights and freedoms that belong to every person in the world, from birth until death (www. equalityhumanrights.com/en/human-rights/what-are-human-rights). They apply regardless of where you are from, what you believe or how you choose to live your life. The Universal Declaration of Human Rights, adopted by the United Nations (UN) in 1948, sets out the basic rights and freedoms that apply to everyone in the world, forming the basis of international human rights laws. The European Convention on Human Rights (ECHR) protects the human rights of people in countries that belong to the Council of Europe. The Convention consists of numbered 'articles' protecting basic human rights (see European Court of Human Rights, 2010). In the UK, these rights are enshrined in the Human Rights Act (1998). Human rights are protected globally by the UN. The Convention on the Rights of Persons with Disabilities was adopted by the UN in 2006. It re-affirms that *all persons* with *all types of disabilities* must enjoy *all human rights* and fundamental freedoms. These rights are protected in the UK, through the Equality Act (formerly the Disability Discrimination Act 1995) which was introduced in 2010. It gives legal protection from discrimination, including age discrimination.

People living with dementia are frequently denied their human rights even when regulations are in place to uphold them. This happens as a result of paternalistic attitudes, lack of knowledge, and an over-emphasis on risk. People with dementia and carers can also find that they have different needs, and as a result, the rights of the person with dementia, as distinct and equally important, can get lost (see, for example, the work of Dementia Alliance www.dementiaallianceinternational.org). In 2015, the

World Health Organization published guidance on human rights and dementia referring to the PANEL principles. These principles deconstruct what a human rights based approach means in practice. PANEL stands for Participation, Accountability, Non-Discrimination and Equality, Empowerment and Legality. Human rights are inextricably linked to both recognising and valuing resilience in others. We can do this by finding ways to maximise participation and demonstrating accountability through resilience-focused practice. This includes: treating people with dementia with the same respect that we treat others; finding space and time for people to tell their stories, in their own way; and empowering people by maximising opportunities for individual resilience to flourish.

Some Things to Keep in Mind

'Resilience' is not a neutral term and cannot be looked at in a vacuum. Choices are made politically about what it is, how it is recognised, and its application. As a result, some people are automatically thought of as vulnerable, or as lacking resilience, or adaptive capacity. The context in which resilience is applied, by whom, and for what outcome is fundamental. Resilience is defined as different things, by different groups, and applied in different ways, to achieve specific outcomes. Human rights and the PANEL approach can ensure that people with dementia are not subject to inconsistent quality of service. As mentioned before, there is a very small body of literature dealing with the subject of resilience and dementia. Further, it is a complex process, which includes the interaction of vulnerability and protective factors, and is context specific, not a fixed state. To this end, level of need or support, or independence are not indicators of resilience. Instead, they can be thought of as the catalyst for a resilience process. This can be difficult to see when traditional views of resilience seem to move us away from this understanding. In the next chapter we will, therefore, look at new concepts and the ways in which they help shape our understanding of a model of resilience for people living with dementia.

CHAPTER 2

Re-Imagining Resilience

New Concepts and Connections

Although attitudes to dementia are changing, organisational responses to people with dementia, carers and care partners remain relatively unchanged. As a result, there is now an urgent need for those working in this field to connect with people living with dementia in new ways. This chapter will explore new concepts that impact on our understanding of dementia and resilience, and those that cause us to stop and think differently about how we organise support and care.

Reserve Capacity and Cognitive Reserve

'Reserve capacity' is a term used to explain how bodily organs function when under stress. It is a subject of great relevance to the prevention of dementia. Why do some people develop dementia as they age and other people don't? It is thought that educational attainment, occupation and mental stimulation, such as learning a second language, all reduce the risk of dementia. Reserve capacity is distinctly about the body's tolerance to dementia and pathological changes to the brain. Cognitive reserve, however, refers to how the brain then maintains a good enough level of functioning where pathological changes do occur, for example, as a result of Alzheimer's disease (Stern, 2012). This has been explained as an emphasis on maintaining tasks and the activities of daily life, rather than reversing a person's cognitive condition. For example, a study by Snowden, in 1997, referred to as the 'Nun Study', revealed that the neuropathology discovered in brains post mortem didn't always correlate with levels of functioning reported during life. Some of the people with dementia in this study functioned better than would have been expected by simply examining the changes or damage to the brain. Cognitive reserve theory posits that the brain finds different ways to respond to loss of function by employing reserves from another area. This capacity for compensation, and flexibility, is thought to develop through the accumulation of skills and knowledge acquired, as a result of complex mental functions and problem solving, over a lifetime. Life experiences, social activities, education and social networks can all potentially contribute to this reserve. In other words, mental and social activity throughout life may facilitate flexible cognitive resources which we can use even when we have dementia. Further, it may also be possible for people who have dementia to retain the capacity *to continue to develop compensation strategies whilst living with dementia*. This appears to go against everything we know about the impact of dementia, functional and neurological decline. However, it opens the door to using reserve capacity to think about resilience, and the rich repository of skills, assets and resources that a person might be able to fall back on. I have referred to this as the Resilience Reserve and it is illustrated in Figure 2.1.

As described above, our Resilience Reserve is a personal repository that each of us has to meet the challenges and demands of life. We build this reserve through our knowledge, skills, experiences, networks, assets and resources. The more that we look to our own reserve in order to meet these challenges successfully, then the more trust we build in ourselves that we can meet future adversities head on and find a way through. But how do we know what tools we have in our personal reserve to respond? Are there resources we have that we could employ that we don't? And can you replenish your Resilience Reserve when you feel overwhelmed by events? Much like the work of Daniel and Wassell in their workbooks on resilience in children (2002a, 2002b, 2002c), I discuss aspects of the resilience reserve in six domains. Each of these can be considered as contributing to the person's ability to respond in times of crisis and reflect the accumulation of resources that we each possess.

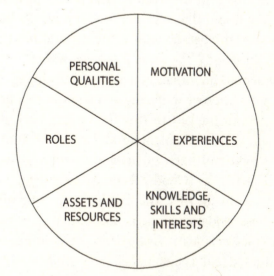

Figure 2.1 The Resilience Reserve

Using these domains we can methodically collect information on a focused topic. It also opens up a dialogue on the range of interventions available to people living with dementia. For example, it is suggested that interventions such as re-ablement, rehabilitation (including exercise) and memory training can promote the further development of the cognitive reserve; or it can help people to use their existing cognitive reserve in different ways, and to better effect (Clare *et al.*, 2010; Clare *et al.*, 2017). Re-ablement means restoring function and function refers to *what you can do*. Moreover, taking part in such activities also appears to promote wellbeing in both the person with dementia and carers. Everyday activities are the important foundations of our lives and who we are, as individuals, within families and within communities. Being unable to undertake these activities can be devastating. Research by Giebel and Sutcliffe (2017) highlighted that most studies into everyday activities and dementia focus on what a person can no longer do; instead, they asked, 'how does this make you feel?' They found that reduced function affects both the wellbeing of the person with dementia and the stress or sense of burden for the carer. However, where the person with dementia can initiate activities of daily living this can significantly improve wellbeing and reduce carer stress.

Despite an interest in this field going back to 2004 (Marshall, 2004), re-ablement and rehabilitation programmes have not been inclusive of people living with dementia generally (Goodwin and Allan, 2019). There are several reasons for this. The first is therapeutic nihilism, that is, there is no cure for dementia, or that all people with dementia lack capacity. As a result, intervention options can be limited to the person, their presenting problems and service input. Sometimes, the person embodies 'the problem of dementia' in the mind of professionals and carers, and practice then focuses on 'the problem of this person'. The concern is that these views lead to continued positioning of people with dementia as having no resilient resources and as being inherently 'hopeless people'. External resources are also a contributing reason for lack of activity in this field, whether it is the assumption that investing time with a person with dementia to improve functioning would be futile, or that it takes an infinite amount of time or resources to provide rehabilitation, or both. This was confirmed in a small Australian study exploring the views of health professionals on the provision of multi-disciplinary rehabilitation for people with dementia (Cations *et al.*, 2019). If we start from the perspective that the person has no resources to build on then these attitudes are more likely. People with dementia are not routinely referred to physiotherapists or audiologists, for example. Dementia is seen as a specific thing that affects the independence of the person and causes a gradual loss of capacity. Adapting to sensory changes, issues with balance, seeking to improve these things, and cope with changes, does not feature as part of routine dementia support at this time (Houston and Christie, 2018), despite the potential benefits to functioning and wellbeing.

Practitioners can also be confused about what re-ablement or rehabilitation looks like for people living with dementia and whose job it is to deliver this. There are 'how to' books and guides that practitioners can access with hints and tips (for example, Kelly and O'Sullivan, 2015; O'Connor *et al.*, 2018; Pool, 2018). Technology also offers opportunities. However, unlike other health conditions, when a person has dementia, the tasks to be addressed through rehabilitation are not always easily articulated. In order to develop a meaningful plan it is necessary to spend time with the person, and then focus on the goals that he or she would like to achieve, and identify the tasks or steps required in order to reach the intended goal. For example, someone might want to continue to cook for the family. A team of allied health professionals, such as occupational therapists, and support staff can then develop a plan through a combination of sequencing, instructions, practice and prompts to make the tasks more manageable and/or safer. The goals are to maintain or improve cognitive function, compensate for memory loss and develop strategies to undertake tasks. The intervention is time limited and goal focused.

Motivation

We also cannot assume that we know what each person's goals are. For example, Beth is 89 years old and lives alone in sheltered housing. Beth's short-term memory isn't good. However, she isn't worried too much about this. Beth gauges the impact of dementia in her life by how well she remembers important people and her emotional connection to them. This is her daily check. She does not remember the day before, or day-to-day events. She keeps detailed notes which she reads over in the morning, and at night, to try and piece together what is happening in the present. On the whole, Beth feels that life is good.

'My memory's not that bad. It's not terrible. I mean I remember my gran and my home and I remember the house and all these things. Well, say I've got a date to be somewhere... I know I won't remember it so I have to write in on the calendar. So if I've got to go to a place, I'll write it down. So I'll not forget! I remember that I forget, you know? Yes, yes. It's not that bad. As long as I can remember way back it's only the last few years that I don't remember... There was nothing really to be done about it, if you know what I mean? I know things aren't going to stay.'

So, for Beth, what motivates her is being able to recollect key people in her life. Managing around the home is not considered important. Beth does not feel that dementia has negatively impacted on her life. In their study of resilience, Forstmeier and Maercker (2008) discussed motivation and motivational skills in relation to resilience in later life, including life with dementia. Motivation and apathy are positioned as opposing ends of a spectrum. They suggest that where a person has clear motivations and is able to act with reference to these, this can minimise the impact of later life as a negative experience. In this study, estimates of mid-life motivational abilities were made using data about people's occupations and occupational performance. This was then used to estimate the motivational reserve that the person may still have access to in older age. They found that there was a possible link between motivational abilities in mid-life and those in later life, and that apathy was associated with lower resilience as we age. Ottmann and Maragoudaki (2015) also identified motivation as essential in the resilience strategies of older people. Motivation is an important domain in our personal Resilience Reserve. Motivations are also extremely personal to us. They are shaped by our unique experiences. It is, therefore, important to remember that dementia and ageing are experienced differently by all of us. Recently, researchers and commentators have turned to intersectionality to explore this.

Intersectionality

Intersectionality (Crenshaw-Williams, 1989) explores the interlocking systems of oppression and power that people experience in their lives. This simply means that we are not all powerful or all powerless as our lives and relationships are complex. So, all older people are not equally dis-advantaged by ill-health, ageism, sexism or racism, to name but a few, as they have different roles, status, financial means, experiences, etc. This is of particular relevance where older people are discussed as a homogeneous group. We still organise services and service responses around this concept, even though, on age alone, this 'group' can consist of people over five different decades from age 60, to the lucky few who are 100 years old and beyond. The application of intersectionality also highlights that one person cannot claim to represent the totality of experiences of a specific group, for example, a white, older woman could not claim to speak for the experiences of all women on the experience of being an *older woman*. This particular person could be in a position of privilege if, for example, they have never experienced poverty or racial discrimination.

Intersectionality reminds us of the individuality of each experience, the importance of identity and power, and the need to think about overlapping experiences of discrimination and acceptance. For example, a study by Hulko (2009) sought the views of eight people about the experience of living with dementia. She found that older people who have experience of coping with oppression in their lives, prior to dementia, may be able to apply this developed resilience to the context of their life with dementia. As a result some people don't think about dementia as a catastrophic event in their life, and instead, experience dementia as just 'one more hurdle' (p.140). In comparison, a person who has enjoyed a position of privilege or status can be devastated by the label of dementia. The lack of experience of adversity may mean that they have less well developed resilience and are less equipped to deal with the stigma and changes in their lives. This was the case with Alan. Alan is 92 years old and a keen golfer. He lives with his wife.

'I didn't know about the dementia until last year. I had gone to hospital for some sort of checks. So, it was quite a few weeks afterwards that I got information via the doctor that I had a slight tendency to dementia. That was the first I'd heard of it, you know? No, not only that but when they told me it was that I never felt any different than I had that day. It was just at the, the surgery, it was a lady doctor who is in charge of the surgery so it was through her that I heard... I was a wee bit depressed when I found that as I always felt so healthy, you know?'

Talking about the complexity of life, and the intersecting experiences we have, of having status in some parts of our lives but not others, facilitates different thinking about both dementia and resilience. An important aspect of this is the relationships that we have with other people in our lives. This is covered in the next topic of interdependence.

Interdependence

Dependence is talked about as an inevitable outcome for people ageing with dementia. Society talks about the burden of old age and certainly 'the burden of cost to society' is everyday language in policy and politics. But what if we thought of dependence differently? What if we thought about the right to be dependent and to be in need of care and support at different points in our lives? Care ethics (Bubeck, 1995; Tronto, 1994) address the complexity of care as an essential human right, a human value, a public policy issue, a function of public bodies and as potentially oppressive in the lives of older and disabled people. This reflects the complexity of our lives where it is possible to both receive care, and at the same time to provide care to others. This change in perspective is essential if we are to think about resilience. Resilience can address the loss of citizenship, and loss of roles, that can occur, through predictable policy and care options for older people. This can, in turn, help us to re-balance rights, status and recognition. If we refresh our perspective on human rights, as the right to be dependent at times, and move to a model of interdependence where we recognise that all of us depend on other people at some points in our life, we can change the dominant discourse. Care must be taken not to confuse 'being independent' with proof of resilience. This conflict around the need to promote independence, and at the same time address risks for people living with dementia, can be seen where independence is discussed as a status that is granted to people living with dementia. This implies that the status of *being dependent* is the expected norm when working with people with dementia. Although practitioners have a duty to protect adults considered to be vulnerable to risk (see for example, the Adult Support and Protection (Scotland) Act, 2007) the starting point for engagement must be the recognition of a person's rights in accordance with the Human Rights Act (1998). Practice must then address risky situations and consider what support the person with dementia needs to promote independence in those areas, or it must evidence where freedoms have to be restricted in accordance with the appropriate legislation. A resilience framework is a useful tool in such necessary discussions. This approach is compatible with citizenship models of dementia, as to approach independence as something to be earned would represent a challenge to realising the resilience of the person with dementia in practice. Re-framing all of our lives within the context of society as consisting of interdependent citizens could be a useful approach. One way to do this is to think about how we age within our communities, neighbourhoods and families.

This re-situates ageing from an individual to a connected experience and can help us to visualise the wealth of assets, and resources, that we already have in our lives, to help ourselves and others.

Asset-Based Approaches

An asset-based approach seeks to positively mobilise the assets, capacities or resources available to a person and/or a community, which could enable individuals to gain more control over their lives and circumstances. Public health policies typically try to identify 'cause and effect' relationships, with interventions designed to interrupt problematic patterns. This has been effective in tackling health problems, such as preventing infection through immunisation. However, for many people, the issues leading to ill-health or ill-being are linked to social, economic and/or environmental circumstances. Assets can be thought of as *individual assets*, for example, motivation, self-esteem, sense of purpose; *community assets*, for example, networks, social capital, sense of being part of a community; and *organisational or institutional assets*, for example, environmental resources for promoting physical health, employment security and opportunities for volunteering, the provision of quality housing, etc. Organisational assets also refer to political and democratic arrangements that are available to individuals to facilitate the roles and responsibilities of citizens, and the structures in place to meet each person's human rights. The process of *asset mapping* is the first step to help individuals and communities recognise resources that could be available to them. Asset mapping is simply a visualisation of the categories listed above. By visualising the assets in your environment you can make better use of them. Problems to be tackled can then be agreed and solutions found through employing these assets.

Salutogenesis

The theory of salutogenesis, which highlights the factors that promote health rather than those that cause disease, is closely linked to asset-based approaches. Salutogenesis emerged within the context of a public health focus on disease, and the causal or risk factors for disease, such as smoking and cancer (Lindstrom and Eriksson, 2006). Antonovsky (1979, 1987, 1991) theorised that stress and disease are always around us. Given this, he was interested in the ways in which people avoided ill-health. He concluded that disease (pathogenesis) and health (salutogenesis) were at opposing ends of a continuum, and considered the factors that prevented a decline towards disease. He concluded that healthier people are able to make sense of their world and they see their lives as meaningful. This is referred to as a 'sense of coherence' (Antonovsky, 1987, p.19). Healthier people also use the resources that they have at their disposal to experience stress but resist illness. Some authors have attempted to align elements of resilience and salutogenesis, for example, Hicks and Conner (2014) have suggested that sense of coherence is simply resilience. However, criticisms of the salutogenic approach appear to challenge this. For example, salutogenesis has failed to take account of people who have limited access to resources as a result of restricted life opportunities, such as poverty (Harrop *et al.*, 2009). It also has a focus on health creation (the literal translation of the term 'salutogenesis'); however, we know that the absence of ill-health does not necessarily equate to wellbeing. For example, salutogenesis had been used by Friedland *et al.* (2001) to explore and explain why not everyone who ages goes on to experience dementia. This research located the absence of dementia as the salutogenic goal, and placed dementia at the disease end of the spectrum as an example of pathogenesis. Dementia is also progressive.

Unlike resilience, salutogenesis has a primary focus on the person in the present, and is less concerned with the contribution that our lived experiences and biography can make (Harrop *et al.*, 2009). People with dementia who experience a threat to their sense of self may experience a loss of mastery and control in their life, or struggle with what these episodes mean within the story of their life. A resilience focus is concerned with how a person could adjust to loss, not the avoidance of loss, as is suggested through the salutogenic model. Taylor (2004) concluded that salutogenesis tends to be associated with those who are well educated and in positions of social or financial privilege, whom Hulko (2009) found might in fact be less resilient when a condition such as dementia is experienced. Both Harrop *et al.* (2009) and Windle (2011) concluded that resilience and salutogenesis were related concepts but distinct discourses.

Co-production

Co-production is where citizens are involved in the creation of public policies and services. It is seen as a move away from a customer/consumer model of services. In order for this to happen we must recognise the skills, knowledge, assets and resources of citizens and acknowledge the inherent power imbalance that exists in transactions between people who use services, and statutory planners, service delivery structures and budget holders. Co-production is distinct from consultation and involvement. It is an authentic communication process where the agenda is set by the people involved, and the ownership of the problem, and the solution, is shared. It relies on making the best use of the skills, assets and resources of people and communities. Stereotypes of people with dementia, and assumptions about what people with dementia can do, can make both co-production and opportunities for resilience less likely, as the person's knowledge and experience acquired throughout their life might be dismissed as irrelevant. However, this can be a missed opportunity. There are now many examples of people with dementia working with and in some cases taking control of international, national and local agendas around dementia (see, for example, the Scottish Dementia Working Group: www.sdwg.org.uk).

Looking more closely at the personal or domestic citizenship aspects of dementia in care work, we often assume responsibility for problem solving. This means undertaking personal care and household tasks for people with dementia. In doing so we fall into predictable care routines and practices which can upset the natural rhythm of people's lives, and can leave people feeling that circumstances are outside their control. Reflecting back on the earlier part of this chapter, this approach makes re-ablement less likely. To be frank, it is the easiest and least expensive option if we do not see the human cost of such service responses. If we take doing the laundry as an example, a person with dementia might need help for the following reasons. He or she might forget to do the laundry, be unable to initiate the task, or it might get done repetitively. The person might not understand how to operate the washing machine, or mix up the contents being washed. Clothing might not be clean or could be washed at the wrong settings. Where there are no prompts or directions to help, or a carer to step in, the situation can deteriorate to the point that clothing worn is dirty, and the person appears dishevelled. It is then often at this point that referrals are made to services as the person's physical appearance suggests that they are not managing. By changing the conversation to one of untapped potential, and the impact on the person's self-image when such referrals are made and tasks are re-allocated, we can begin to see a role for resilience. Resilience is fostered by a sense of having control over one's circumstances, as we will discover later. How often do our interventions take this away from people through the support that we provide? Instead, focus on finding out the exact details as to why domestic arrangements break down (moving from a 'because of dementia' approach) and, with the person, testing the ways in which tasks and roles can be restored with the right support. We should only make alternative arrangements when this is not possible. This is the foundation of facilitating resilience in practice.

Summary

In conclusion, resilience doesn't mean invulnerability to disease or hardship; quite the contrary. Resilience can, in fact, be the experience of oppression and hardship but finding a way to live, to improve your wellbeing, and to function despite these circumstances. Resilience also isn't just about thriving or independence. It can be about depending on others and others being dependent on us, reflecting the interconnectedness of life. We can think about this as overlapping lives and overlapping experiences of life. We don't always understand what motivates people, but we can learn more if we listen to the stories we tell each other about who we are, what we have done and what we want to do. Thinking differently about dementia and resilience means reflecting on the ways in which current practice is shaped around grouping *older people* and *people with dementia* together. We also tend to assume that dementia is the worst thing that has happened to the person. It isn't always the worst thing and not everyone has a bad experience of life with dementia. We have to keep an open mind about how people feel, and what motivates them. For some, it is the caring responsibilities that they have for others, for some it might be to live life with as little change as possible despite dementia. Most important of all, sometimes it is those people who appear to have the fewest resources in life who might emerge as the most resilient.

CHAPTER 3

The Experience of Threat and Dementia

The Possibility of Resilience

Although not everyone with dementia can be resilient, there is the possibility of resilience despite, or perhaps because of, dementia. However, a person with dementia can find their actions being misunderstood or misinterpreted. Take John, for example. John's family found that he was regularly misplacing items in the home. His family had to buy him a new remote control for his television on several occasions. John was embarrassed about this and made up his mind not to lose the latest one. Alas, this one was lost too and was eventually found in the fridge by his daughter. John's family were worried. Surely, this new development confirmed Dad's worsening condition. However, what no one knew was that when John lost things he had a habit of stopping, and making a cup of tea, and he would have a good think about where the missing item might be. John also liked milk in his tea, and so, at an earlier point, he had decided to put the remote control in the fridge because he knew he would find it next to the milk eventually. John had devised his own solution to this problem to avoid future embarrassment in his relationship with his daughter, but because he couldn't share his reasoning or explanation, or remember having done this, it was labelled as just another symptom of his worsening dementia.

In trying to understand resilience from the perspective of a person with dementia, both dementia and ageing can be considered as life adversities. This happens as relationships change which, in turn, can affect how we think about ourselves. Sometimes we can feel diminished in once comfortable, predictable family and social situations. The result of this is that people with dementia can experience distress and upset to their sense of wellbeing. Resilience is the process of regaining a sense of wellbeing as the person responds to these emotional changes and challenges. We can recognise these emotional threats and adaptations if we know what we are looking for. So, the issue in John's example isn't the safe keeping of the remote control but the impact of the changing relationship between John and his daughter which is highlighted by the situation. This can be thought of as losing one's domestic citizenship (Bartlett, 2016). This occurs where a person's role and status in the home, and in the context of home life, is diminished as a result of dementia. This isn't a deliberate act in most cases. John's daughter, for example, is worried about him and wants to help.

Within wider society, reports on social attitudes to dementia over the recent past (for example, ScotCen Social Research and the Life Changes Trust, 2015, 2018) have found that, although a substantial number of respondents have positive views about people with dementia, stigmatising views are also held. This includes the view that having dementia is something to be ashamed of. The person ageing with dementia could be described as having attributes associated with an 'undesirable state of being'. Stigma in this case can be considered as a symbolic rejection of ageing and disease. It can also be argued that stigma is present in the language used to discuss the growing numbers of people ageing with dementia, where words such as *epidemic* and *burden* are used to stress the need to act quickly in delaying the onset of dementia (Department of Health, 2012; Wilson and Fearnley, 2007; World Health Organization, 2012). Materialistic arguments perpetuate the discourse, first explored by De Beauvoir in 1977, that older people (with dementia) are considered as a socio-economic and health burden as they no longer contribute to the economy. This argument gives no consideration to the previous contributions made by people throughout their lives, or the contributions made by caring for grandchildren and voluntary work that many people are engaged in (Joint Improvement Team and NHS Health Scotland, 2014). Instead, it can perpetuate existing systems of care and support which see many people with dementia moving into institutional care (Prince *et al.*, 2013). Stigma can therefore be used as a mechanism to maintain the status quo in situations of power and inequality, with the literature asserting that many people can internalise these negative messages which then shape personal and public identities (Batsch and Mittelman, 2012; Gove *et al.*, 2016). If stigma is to be addressed and challenged then resilience may offer a helpful perspective.

Identity and Dementia

In relation to dementia there is ongoing debate about what identity means when aspects of the person are assumed to have changed. There are questions as to whether identity can continue to exist and in what ways (Caddell and Clare, 2010; Hughes *et al.*, 2006). The development of identity over the lifespan was explored through the work of Erikson (1965, 1968, 1980), who referred to identity as 'ego identity'. Erikson proposed that identity continues to develop beyond childhood and identified eight distinct stages where this occurs over the life cycle. The final stage of 'ego integrity versus despair' describes a period of self-reflection where each person assesses the contributions and achievements of his or her life, resulting in a sense of completeness or despair. Similarly, Butler (1963) used the phrase 'life review' to describe the stage of reflection and making sense of one's life story in older age. Critics of this approach to thinking about ageing (e.g. McCrae and Costa, 1997) highlighted the lack of reference to the individual, existing structural inequalities, issues of power and the impact of each person's unique circumstances. Instead, experiences of ageing are discussed as though they are universal, and as a result, poor experiences of ageing are attributed as the fault of the individual. This can lead to assumptions that all persons living with dementia will have a poor experience of ageing.

Symbolic Interactionist Perspectives of Identity and Dementia

Goffman (1959) used the theatre as a metaphor for present-ations of the self in social interaction. People within interaction were considered as social actors and Goffman considered them to have both off-stage and on-stage personas, which Wolfe (1997) stated were used to represent the distinctions between private and public identities. The importance of this distinction is that the private self contains elements that each person chooses not to reveal to others. Goffman considered that the public self was a 'collaborative manufacture' (1959, p.253) which we achieve through adopting a selected or preferred representation of self which he called a 'personal front' (p.24), the purpose being to manage other people's impressions of us. Caddell and Clare (2011, p.198) discussed the 'private self' and the 'interpersonal self' (p.200) in their model of identity in dementia which is similar to Goffman's description of private and public identities. People who have dementia can find that they have little say over how other people view them after their diagnosis becomes public. However, if we accept that citizenship is an active process where a person with dementia achieves recognition and status as 'citizen' through their everyday interactions (Barnes *et al.*, 2004), new ways of understanding dementia are needed as a person's dementia progresses, and the nature of interactions with others changes. But, let us take a minute to examine why this change occurs and what the underlying processes might be.

Human beings observe and assess the world, categorising the people and objects they encounter relative to themselves. We are, therefore, constantly defining the things we interact with. We categorise people we meet as to how we know them, for example, as a family member or a stranger. We might categorise further through observational criteria, for example, height or eye colour, and so on. We also prioritise those people and things within our environment that are important to us. Our interactions with an employer, for example, may cause us to present ourselves in a more favourable light. Finally, we derive meaning from our interactions with others by constantly interpreting what is said, and how the other person acts towards us. In this way we apply our own meanings to every interaction and in turn are shaped though our interactions with others (Charon, 1992). This emphasis on the realisation of identity, or our sense of self in relation to other people, is grounded in symbolic interactionism (Stryker, 1968). This perspective focuses on social interaction as a catalyst for meaning in everyday life. Charon (1992) advised that there are five main components. First, that individuals are considered as 'dynamic, changing actors' (p.27). Second, society is considered as consisting of individuals engaged in social interaction. Third, that people use both the physical self and the mind to interact with others. Fourth, that people consist of many versions of self that emerge in unique interactions with other people, and finally that reality or 'truth is arrived at through interaction and it is also transformed in the process of interaction' (p.28). So, what does this mean for a person living with dementia?

The Spoiled Identity

This perceived loss of recognition or acquiring a new unwanted and spoiled identity (Goffman, 1963) of 'de-mentia sufferer' can impact on the wellbeing of the person con-cerned. Therefore, it is reasonable to conclude that the preservation of a cherished image of oneself (identity) or sense of self, in the face of the emotional challenges of dementia and life with dementia, can be achieved through resilience. This can be thought of as the balance between the statement, 'I am me' and the question, 'Am I me?' and in the experience of dementia this can be expressed as an 'identity continuum' which visualises the act of maintaining a sense of self. This is represented in Figure 3.1.

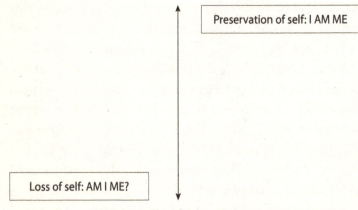

Figure 3.1 The Identity Continuum

We will now take a look in some detail at the different ways that threats to the sense of self can be expressed.

'See, it's my only sort of comeback'

Dora is an 89-year-old woman. She lost a son when he was nine years old to pneumonia and has an adopted son. Her husband passed away ten years ago. Dora is an active member of her church. She has been living with dementia for three years. She also has breathing difficulties and mobility issues. As a result she is now in receipt of round-the-clock care.

> 'You'll need to forgive me as I can't remember. My memory is not what it used to be. And even nowadays I have to write in a calendar and they laugh at me and they tell me, if they come in and tell me anything special I put it down in the calendar. That's stood me in good stead many a time because they say, "Mum, I told you that already" and I say, "right you are, darling, if you told me that it will be down on the calendar" and they go, "Oh, mum, I was sure I had told you." That is my only comeback. Because what would get me is they would say, "I told you that already" and I would know that they had not told me… Oh, and they say you know and say, "Oh I was sure I had told you." See, it's my only sort of comeback in a way to keep me right.'

Dora appears to place her memory loss within a competition narrative: a competition between herself and other members of the family. Dementia appears to threaten Dora's identity as a person who can provide factual, accurate information and all this implies about her competence and status in the family. This is how Dora rejects the spoiled identity (Goffman, 1963) of a person with dementia. This offers a valuable insight into Dora's experience of the domestic sphere of citizenship.

'You'll have to get a carer'

Alan talks about hearing that he had dementia and what this means for him in his relationship with his wife.

> 'So I had to accept that I had dementia so I started to try and get some information about what it was all about. And you know "you'll have to get a, a carer to look after you for a lot of the time", so my wife is really my carer.'

Alan is keen to share how unlike a 'person with dementia' he is. In particular, he discusses how his diagnosis had been at odds with his sense of feeling well. Alan also uses the opportunity to describe in detail his experience of the diagnostic process, and he reflects on whether his wife is now his carer. This is an example of the dichotomy of identity on sameness and selfhood (Ricoeur, 1992) as Alan contemplates what being a person with dementia now means for him. The fundamental question for Alan appears to be, 'Am I the same or now changed?' Taylor (2018, p.20) tells us that this is resilience in action as resilience occupies the spaces between 'being' and 'becoming'.

Threats to identity are revealed within the context of relationships with others for many people with dementia. These relationships are often examined for evidence of sameness, offering a mirror in which one can see the self through the eyes of others. Where evidence of change is found in these relationships this appears to be experienced as a threat by some. People living with dementia can experience threats in relation to changing roles, changing status within families and changing relationships with partners and children. This confirms the role of others in creating and threatening the personal and public self. This is demonstrated in this further example from Alan.

'It's cast up to you'

'Being told about dementia didn't affect the family. Well, I don't think it did, at least they never said and they haven't started avoiding me or anything like that, often though in argument with my wife she'll raise it she'll say, "well you've got dementia!" Well, one night there we were both sitting talking… And she said to me, "what have you done with the coaster, you were the last person using it and I've not got dementia." So sometimes that's cast up to you. How does this make you feel? Oh, not very good.'

Alan states that nothing had changed in his relationship with his family but then recalls how dementia now features in arguments with his wife. This appears to threaten his perspective on his role and identity within the family. This is an example of malignant social positioning (Sabat, 2006). Alan does not challenge his wife in the story he tells. However, his choice of words tells the listener that he feels *accused* of having dementia, and this then provides an insight into Alan thinking that his wife might blame him, either for his diagnosis, or for his behaviour. Alan might feel that his interactions with his wife are less meaningful as a result of dementia (Johannessen and Moller, 2013; Sorensen *et al.*, 2008). This could be an example of a micro-injustice (Bartlett, 2016) within the home, and in the context of his relationship with his wife. It could also be an example of epistemic injustice (Fricker, 2007), where a person is excluded from the creation and co-creation of knowledge, as others perceive they have nothing to offer or are unable to make a contribution. Young *et al.* (2019, p.76) explain that people with dementia experience epistemic injustice when they are 'denied their right to speak, to be heard and to be believed'. We also saw this in Dora's example, of keeping a record of appointments on her calendar so that she could pre-empt such injustices.

'I'm quite under control'

We met Ellen earlier. Ellen's focus is her family and social life.

> 'My daughter organised home helps. And it wasn't as if the place was hanging with cobwebs or whatever. My daughter thought that someone coming in might do me good as she is working, so whether it's needed or not someone comes in. I'm quite under control. I'm very lucky with my neighbours round here and I am not on their doorstep all the time – if I were I probably wouldn't be liked. No, I'm very fortunate if I need someone.'

This example, as told by Ellen, demonstrates tensions, and threats to sense of self, experienced by a person with dementia, within the context of the care provided by others. Ellen considers herself to be independent. Being in receipt of support can affect your sense of self and the person you believe yourself to be. Meléndez and Pitarque (2018) describe a tendency to 'magical thinking' in people with more advanced dementia. By this they mean that what a person thinks about a situation, problem or solution isn't always based in the reality of the situation. But is this relevant?

Of course, where risks are involved practitioners are required to delve deeper rather than focus on surface stories. Dementia brings a person's competence into question as judgements are made about what 'people with dementia' can do. Conversation re-framed as narrative reveals stories and story content rich with expressions of identity. The stories people tell help us to understand their worries and concerns, as well as what is important to them. This is important as people living with dementia can be thought of by others as passive or non-contributing in interpersonal exchanges. Instead, people with dementia have knowledge to share if we are ready to listen, providing an insight into who they are (sense of self) or aspire to be known as (personal front). In the next chapter we will explore the delicate balance of holding on to a sense of self and living life with dementia.

CHAPTER 4

Holding on to a Sense of Self

In order to think about resilience in the lives of people with dementia we need to think differently about dementia. In this chapter we will introduce the idea of survival: survival of self and preservation of our identities in the face of dementia. This can offer new insights into the experience of adapting and adjusting to the different challenges of dementia. I will then develop this further to help us think about how we can visualise resilience.

Dementia and Survival

Lifton (1993) advised that a survivor is one who has encountered death literally, or figuratively. This can result in feelings of separation from individuals, communities and principles; of disintegration (of falling apart or the fear of falling apart); and of paralysis, stasis or immobility, which the person must adjust to or overcome. People with dementia have advised that they feel increasingly disconnected and isolated as dementia progresses. Many people disengage from their communities, families and friends for fear of losing face or find that the people that they know avoid their company. Family roles can be eroded as relationships change along with the dementia trajectory. Each person with dementia could potentially be engaged in a process of continual adjustments, no matter how small, where they adjust to these changes and their life with dementia, even when they are unable to remember or communicate the details. The importance of the everyday is again visible here. Alan shares his experience.

> 'No, I don't feel any different but I didn't find out very much. But I was talking to a chap the other day at the day care place and I said to him I have dementia and he said so have I. And of course his brother had it and he was worse, it got very, very difficult for his mother to handle him, but he was alright or at least he seemed alright. I don't think I'm too difficult to handle.'

Alan rejects any assumptions we might make about him or his behaviour through the label of being 'a person with dementia'. He describes what he believes to be the attributes of someone with dementia, in order that he can demonstrate how different he is from this. The inclusion of others can act as a means of persuasion, of persuading the self and others of a particular point of view, in order that your sense of self can survive despite the changes of dementia. Alan has a friend who has dementia, who like him, is surprised at his diagnosis. He also tells us about an 'out of control' person with dementia. This is possibly revealing Alan's fears about what dementia might mean, that is, to be out of control or changed. It also tells us that people with dementia are ordinary, everyday people living life and finding a way to make sense of the positon that they now find themselves in. This reflects the struggle between sameness and selfhood (Ricoeur, 1992) that we discussed in the previous chapter.

Application of the survivor identity offers an opportunity to re-frame and re-define the actions of people with dementia. Some people might find that they struggle with the changes that dementia brings. There is currently a tension between the image of living well with dementia and the experiences of people who would describe themselves as suffering as a result of dementia. For those people who want to speak of *suffering* with dementia, this does not negate survival. It just indicates an absence of wellbeing. In this case survival might be even more relevant. Importantly, although a person has dementia, survival doesn't have to focus on this. In this example from Lorna, who is a social worker with a local authority team, she comments on a woman that she is working with who had survived the death of her youngest child. The event had understandably had a devastating impact on this person's life but had not defined her.

> 'She wants to impress upon you that she's had difficulties in her life but she's coping. She's come out the other end and that's all part of her resilience. These traumatic incidents have, she advises, made her very strong and I would agree with that. Well, all these things could have broken other people.'

Radden and Fordyce (2006) clarified that survival for a person with dementia is not about having to evidence that you are the same to other people. Instead, survival of some aspect of self may entitle us to 'pronounce some degree of survival between the earlier person that we knew and the much changed person with dementia we now encounter' (p.78). Jaworska (1997) considered that there is evidence of survival where the person with dementia continues to value the same things in his or her life, even where they are unable to remember details of this life. We place so much emphasis on presence and being present in today's culture. This 'hyper presence' is demonstrated in social media culture where we can engage 24/7, with people from around the world, sharing aspects of our lives and debating the issues of the moment. Being unable to demonstrate 'presence' can be taken as evidence that the person is no longer there. However, a different sense of self may be emerging that the person concerned finds comfort in. Reassuring memories, and relationships from another age: a sense of continuity with another part of one's life. This is often viewed as the person 'slipping away' where it seems incongruent with our idea of the present and being present. It may, therefore, be more appropriate to refer to the person as *surviving* rather than as *survivor* as dementia is a continual process of change. Mitchell (2018) explores this to great effect in her book *Somebody I Used to Know*. This is an example of holding on to self through narrative and story.

The Narrative Self

Our unique sense of self, it is theorised, is achieved through the active creation of a 'personal story of which the subject stands as author' (Radden and Fordyce, 2006, p.73). This is known as our narrative self. Our identity is preserved through this telling and re-telling of stories of self. And you thought you were just talking or sharing a conversation! Reissman (2008, p.8) stated that identities are simply stories people tell themselves and others about who they are (and who they are not). Resilience is realised through relationships with others and relationships develop through the sharing of our stories. In the example below, author Wendy Mitchell, who is also living with dementia, shares her experience.

> 'I love walking in the Lake District where walking shoes are essential. Until recently, I've managed in a fashion to tie my own shoe laces. On my last visit, however, I woke to the fog that frequently descends on people with dementia and couldn't tie them. I could no longer work out that simple action. Many would consider this to be a loss, but then, then, online, I discovered "no tie shoelaces". I no longer have the stress of whether I'll be able to tie my laces and have the embarrassment of having to ask someone else to tie them. I can carry on being like everyone else and wearing my walking shoes.'

Here we can see that Wendy sets the scene for the listener that she loves to be outdoors in the Lake District in England. We know from the details that she provides that she goes there regularly and that she has on occasion had problems with her shoe laces, and one morning couldn't tie her laces at all. What this means is that Wendy would then have to accept defeat and forego her walks, or have someone help her with this, which she could have found disabling (not to mention embarrassing). Wendy conveys that she experienced a problem but rather than give up a much loved activity she is able to find a solution. Her resilience is revealed through the listener as they engage with the story and find their own meaning in it.

Realising resilience in stories and relationships is dependent on three factors. First, that practitioners and carers are able to recognise reflections of identity within the everyday stories told by people with dementia, such as Wendy's story about the Lake District. Second, that we can understand the significance of these reflections within a resilience context, and finally, that this concept of 'the resilience of the person with dementia' is incorporated into a wider social understanding of every person that is unique to their own situation.

Each person's life is a rich mix of factors often referred to as risk and protective factors. Rather than increasing vulnerability, ageing can be a strength in the development of resilience. If you think about it, growing older is the only way to gain a long-term perspective on self. The personal, reflective stories that we share, throughout our lives and about our lives, help us to understand ourselves in the context of adversity: how we react, the things that upset us, what we can do to protect ourselves from pain and upset. We know ourselves well. We then spend our lives presenting ourselves to others through talking about our lives and our circumstances. This can be described as another construct of citizenship: narrative citizenship. Baldwin (2008), discussing the concept of narrative citizenship, argued that we are engaged in citizenship simply through the stories we tell about ourselves and our lives, using these to position ourselves relative to others in society. However, this in itself does not necessarily result in rights being recognised, or power for the individual concerned, as stories, such as those told by people with dementia, can be marginalised by others. The narratives of more powerful individuals can then dictate the nature of citizenship and the narratives of the less powerful can remain hidden. Put simply, do we listen when people with dementia speak? If stories of self, or narratives, provide the foundation for resilience to be revealed, then there must be cues or signs. After all, we all share stories but we are not all resilient. There are, therefore, two key components of stories that help us to recognise the potential for resilience and these are *narrative openness* and *autobiographical reasoning*. Narrative openness is described by Randall *et al.* (2015) as a willingness to share expressions of one's self, life, thoughts and views. Autobiographical reasoning is reflecting on scenarios and outcomes in the context of your life story. This can be thought of as the times when you might give the younger version of yourself some advice to do things differently. A scenario lots of us might muse over! This also places a different emphasis on activities such as reminiscence and life story work. Might these be opportunities to explore narrative openness and autobiographical reasoning as part of a resilience approach? Although ageing offers insights into our sense of self over time, resilience can also fade over time. Have you ever looked back on your younger self and wondered how you managed to cope with a difficult problem and been unsure if you could now? Researchers discuss resilience as changing or evolving as we age, with some people becoming more resilient in certain circumstances, as they have a lifetime of experiences to refer to (Allen *et al.*, 2011), whilst other people associate ageing with loss and uncertainty, losing trust in themselves and their abilities. In essence, we are complicated and our lives are complicated. This is reflected in discussions of vulnerability and strengths.

Vulnerability, Risk and Protective Factors

Resilience is a complex interaction of vulnerability, risk and protective factors. These words are used frequently in practice and by professionals in their work with people with dementia, so let's spend a few moments looking at them in some more detail.

Protective factors act as a buffer in the face of adversity. This means that protective factors can lessen the emotional impact of challenging events and situations. As a result, where we cannot remove or reduce the adversity we should promote protective factors. *Protective factors make us more resilient in the face of adversity.* When these buffers aren't sufficient to cushion us from adversity our emotional balance is upset. One of the ways in which we work through resolving this upset is by looking to our personal reserves to find the right tools, to restore our sense of wellbeing and reduce stress and anxiety. We also reach out to others for support where they have resources we need. We do this whenever we speak to people about our worries and problems. Formal supports can also be thought of in this way. The next chapter will focus on this.

Vulnerability can be described as the point where a person's capacity to respond to a challenging situation or an event falls below the threshold needed to respond. Think of it as the point where the person has no reserves to fall back on, or cannot find the right tools to fit the situation that they find themselves in. Where a person is described as 'vulnerable' this means that they are at an increased risk of reduced wellbeing or harm. Vulnerability and resilience can be thought of as opposing ends of a spectrum and risk determines where each person falls on this continuum, and the likelihood of increasing vulnerability. We will return to the subject of risk later to explore this in more detail.

In summary, vulnerability factors increase the likelihood of a negative outcome and protective factors decrease this likelihood. Vulnerability and resilience can be visualised as two ends of a continuum. I refer to this as the risk continuum. This is shown in Figure 4.1.

The preservation of a preferred sense of self is, therefore, more likely where protective factors outweigh vulnerability factors. The matrix in Figure 4.2 explains the theoretical relationship between the identity and risk continuums.

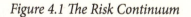

Resilience: protective factors decrease the likelihood of negative outcomes and promote better than expected outcomes.

Vulnerability: risk factors increase the likelihood of negative outcomes.

Figure 4.1 The Risk Continuum

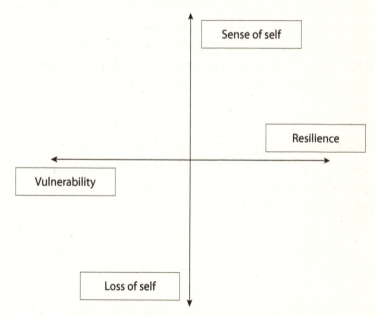

Sense of self

Resilience

Vulnerability

Loss of self

Figure 4.2 The Experience of Dementia Matrix

But what are these vulnerability and protective factors? Are there specific topics that we can focus on to gain insights into the behaviours and actions of people living with dementia? That is what we will explore in the next chapter.

Summary

As we have stated throughout this discussion, people are complex. We each have to make sense of our lives and relationships in order to gain some perspective on self. This enables us to state with confidence 'this is me' and to keep in mind a consistent self-image. We also represent this sense of self to others through our stories, conversations and everyday interactions. This give practitioners a wealth of information about the people that we work with, what makes us tick, and the things that we value in our lives. It also gives us an insight into the infrastructure of people, places and things that help us to retain a sense of wellbeing as we live our lives despite the challenges that we face. Dementia is a unique experience where a person's ability to confidently state 'this is me' can be challenged by their own doubts, but also through the responses of people in their lives who might see the 'dementia' before the person. A resilience framework that recognises all of these component parts of life with dementia is the first step to realising the potential in people's lives. The following chapter will look at this in more detail.

CHAPTER 5

Protective Factors in Action

In this chapter I will explore protective factors in more detail and provide examples of them in action.

Buffers in the Face of Adversity

Protective factors act as buffers in the face of adversity. The more protective factors that the person has, the more resilient they are likely to be, as they act as a cushion in the face of adversity, reducing the impact on the wellbeing of the individual concerned. Conversely, vulnerability factors may increase the impact of adversity, causing emotional distress and anxiety, and make it difficult for a person to respond and adapt. With regard to dementia, protective factors fall under three main headings:

- *sense of connectedness* with others

- *sense of mastery and control* over situations and events

- *meaning making* opportunities.

Connectedness is achieved through personal relationships with the people, places and things in our lives. These relationships should be rewarding and contribute to our sense of wellbeing. As explained before, if identity is shaped and reinforced through the stories we tell others about ourselves, then connectedness has a central role in this. Connectedness includes feeling part of a family, group or community, knowing that there is someone out there who is thinking of you, or is there to fall back on, and importantly, that someone would miss you if you weren't there.

Mastery and control refers to a person's sense of competence and efficacy in a situation: the feeling that in any situation you know what to do, are able to take action, and that this will result in a change or have an impact. This also includes how we are able to influence within our network, and being able to mobilise assets and harness knowledge and skills, to achieve maximum impact.

Meaning making refers to the way in which we make sense of our experiences and interactions with others, and understanding the dynamic nature of our worlds and where dementia fits. We can use these categories within the resilience matrix to identify the protective factors (or buffers) and to identify potential vulnerabilities (see Figure 5.1).

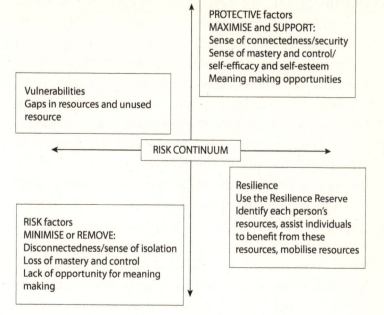

Figure 5.1 The Dementia Resilience Matrix

A Sense of Connectedness

A sense of connectedness is associated with attachment theory (Bowlby, 1980, 1982, 1988). Attachment theory explains the comfort that we derive from close relationships, the mother–child bond being the primary attachment in most cases. In childhood, secure, reliable attachment figures provide a safe base from which to explore the world and to return to in times of ill health or stress (Daniel and Wassell, 2002a). Positive attachments throughout life are, however, important. They provide a source of comfort and assistance to the individual in times of need. We don't have to be in the company of the important people in our lives for them to be meaningful. Sometimes, simply knowing that there is someone, somewhere, thinking about us can make all the difference. The quality of the attachment is also important. We have to be engaged in rewarding relationships which promote our sense of self and our self-esteem. By comparison, relationships which make us feel under-valued, or relationships which are harmful, can have a negative impact on wellbeing. The people in our lives (our attachments) are no less important when we have dementia. Nelis *et al.* (2014) undertook a systematic review looking at attachment in people with dementia and their caregivers. They found that attachment *behaviours* were evident. By this they simply mean that the person with dementia called for, or looked for, an important person in their life, often a parent, even when this person had passed away. This seems self-explanatory. If dementia causes anxiety or uncertainty it is a natural response to seek out a loving parent or partner for comfort. We also know that many people can become confused about the present day and can become anxious if they are looking for a child, not understanding that their son or daughter is now an adult. So, attachment is an important construct.

In a study undertaken by Hedman *et al.* (2013) some people with dementia were aware of previous relationships changing when the other person knew they had dementia. Interactions were experienced as less rewarding and the person was aware that their contribution to the relationship did not appear to be valued. Earlier, we heard from Alan who discussed his changing relationship with his wife. Here he expresses the importance of the relationship to him.

'I try and remember where I left the thing and I try and cope. I decide well I've got it I must cope with it, what else can you do except jump off a bridge or something. Life goes on. Absolutely and I have a wife to worry about, better worrying about her than me… My wife and I go to bed early and put a disc on…and you feel all is right with the world. You know you're together, you're safe. The house is locked up. Cosy… Well, I manage to cope with dementia by going to this place up on the road once a week and talking about it. I don't mind people knowing, well, not really until they ask. But, I just told them I had dementia but I haven't told the newspaper boy and he delivers the news every day.'

Alan's story reveals the worry he feels about dementia. However, he describes a sense of comfort, security and a release from thinking about having dementia, through a focus on his wife and his home. This appears to provide him with respite from his worries about dementia. His struggle to adjust to his dementia is evident in this section. For example, Alan equates coping with striving to remember. This is, of course, not a strategy that he can use in the long term as short-term memory loss is inevitable. Alan also discusses telling other people that he has dementia. He retains a sense of control over his dementia by choosing to whom to disclose amongst his connections. Alan also wishes for others to see him as the same despite his dementia. To this end, the importance of the newspaper boy is interesting, and is a great example of a detail that in traditional assessments would probably go unnoticed. He is not part of Alan's family. He and Alan only have a single daily interaction. However, he is significant to Alan precisely because of their daily interactions. He may be a barometer for Alan to test whether he is 'doing okay' (Harris, 2008) beyond immediate family or the circle of people that he chooses to disclose his dementia to. He is, therefore, an important connection for Alan between his pre-dementia life and now.

This detailed exploration of the protective factors also tells us lots about the risks. The risk factors have a thematic relationship with the protective factors. For example, they follow the same key themes of connectedness, sense of mastery and control, and opportunities for making sense of life with dementia. For example, an absence of connectedness, that is, disconnection and/or a sense of isolation would be an associated risk, so avoiding loneliness in later life and maintaining social activities and hobbies where possible is key. However, being alone is not the same as being lonely. So, the aim is not to keep the person in constant contact with other people. Instead, rewarding friendships and connections which validate the person's sense of self are important. Not all relationships are positive. Relationships where the person is subjected to a continual stream of negative messages pose a risk to wellbeing and increase the likelihood of low self-esteem and self-stigma. This includes abusive relationships. People with dementia can have their human rights ignored and some people are subject to emotional, physical and financial abuse by people they know well. Self-stigma can result in avoiding people and places that you know for fear of being 'caught out' in a social situation. As well as this, disconnectedness from self, and from the person that you believe yourself to be, can occur when valued roles, responsibilities and relationships change or are lost.

Mastery and Control

Mastery and control means knowing that we are able to influence the people and events around us. They incorporate elements of self-esteem and self-efficacy in that we have realistic confidence in ourselves, and our skills, and we can use these skills to take action and avoid ill-being and upset. Self-esteem is about knowing your own worth and also extends to respecting the worth of others. It is closely associated with our sense of self and can be influenced by our appearance or body image, the reactions of others to us, and our satisfaction with our life and relationships in general. So it's a complex mix of internal and external factors. For example, a person with dementia might hold a positive view of themselves as capable but this might not be validated by other people in their network who might see them as vulnerable.

Another issue that affects self-esteem is *social competence*. Social competence refers to effectiveness in social situations and this is dependent on how you act in public situations (your social skills), your understanding of and ability to adapt to social nuances and how you are regarded by others. Dementia can result in the loss of social skills. It can affect your ability to pick up on social cues, and can also mean that you are more sensitive to environmental and social triggers. For example, raised voices could make a person feel anxious or guilty even where the person with dementia is not the subject. Social competence is closely linked to positioning.

Positioning

We discussed positioning earlier. It concerns the position that we take relative to other people when we interact with them. This means we assign categories to the people we meet, for example, friend, boss, etc. and we respond to them in this role. We also assign an identity to ourselves in these interactions and respond within these interactions accordingly. Simply, we are different in the company of close family than we are in a meeting with our boss. We make judgements about people, and where we already hold an opinion about another person, such as someone with dementia, we can interpret what they say to us (their stories) using the meanings that we have already assigned to them (Berger and Luckman, 1966). People with dementia can, therefore, be positioned by others as passive, incompetent and vulnerable. Sabat (2006) stated that this can erase the identity of a person with dementia, where no opportunity arises for the person to challenge this positioning, or challenges are misinterpreted as symptoms of confusion and dementia (Kelly, 2010). This lack of opportunity to challenge can then negatively impact on the person's sense of self.

A person with dementia can use positioning strategies within their own stories to resist this daily malignant positioning. Each person can potentially shape new stories in keeping with their sense of self and preferred public persona. I have identified three distinct positioning approaches that a person with dementia can employ. These are: rejecting the positioning of self by others within stories; re-positioning of self through stories; and positioning dementia within stories of the relational self with others. If we can recognise the strategies that we hear in these stories they can be important indicators of resilience.

Rejecting and Re-Positioning Self Within Stories

Alan tells the story of leaving his golf club.

'Did I join a club when I moved over here from Edinburgh? No, I didn't bother. No. I gave my clubs away to my son-in-law, but maybe one of these bright days he might want to have a full round with me which I would like. I don't, I was very disappointed I had to give up golf and motoring. I don't know if I really gave it up… I moved here as I had family here, not far from here… Well it wasn't about the dementia.'

Alan informs the listener that he has not joined a new club and that he has, in fact, given his golf clubs to his son-in-law. Giving away his clubs is a pivotal part of this story. The golf clubs might be a symbol of Alan's previous life, and all that golf means to him, for example, fitness and public recognition of his skills. The story of giving his clubs away might be Alan's way of indicating this new period of his life. He shares emotional insights into how disappointed he is at giving up driving and golf. This is an example of narrative openness (Randall *et al.*, 2015). Alan provides us with insights into these recent losses. There is also a *point of reflection* signalled by the statement, 'I don't know if I really gave it up'. He concludes insisting that he did not have to give up golf and driving because of dementia, but rather due to lifestyle factors.

For Dora, driving is a skill that she is proud of and it is associated with being needed and valued. She was an advanced driver and was known as such within her family and community. Driving was an important part of her public identity.

'And when I go out a run, I love driving and I passed my advanced driving test. That's my daughter's car. They won't let me drive now. A couple of the parish pastors would say to me at different times "Dora, are you going to church this year?" And right away I knew what was coming. "Well, were you wanting a ride?" "Well, if you don't mind as it means I can leave the car for my wife." So many a time I took the ministers around in my car! I used to love going a run in my car and that's the thing I miss but in my heart I knew. They asked me to read something and I couldn't see it and I thought, "I'm not driving." So they didn't stop me, I stopped myself. The minute I knew I couldn't read a sign I stopped myself. No way would I

put anyone's life in danger but I feel God has been good
to me.'

Dora uses the phrase, 'They won't let me drive now.' However, as her story progresses, she then re-positions herself
as the person who made the decision about her own
competence to drive. Dora does not refer to dementia as
the reason why these decisions were taken. Instead, she is
very specific that her driving stopped because of failing
eyesight. Her decision not to include dementia could be
considered an active act of omission in order to distance
herself from the identity of 'person with dementia'. Dora
uses this opportunity to re-position herself from being
passive to being the active person in control of the situation.
She then re-affirms her personal identity as a good, moral
person and ends with a reference to God. This appears to
be how Dora would prefer to be seen by others.

These adjustments in relation to everyday losses and
routine activities, in order to preserve identities, are
important, revealing the association between dementia
and loss of recognition. In these examples the person does
not simply accept loss, but instead re-interprets the loss
through the act of re-positioning. A sense of mastery over
the situation was established by moving self from passive
to active, so loss of recognition can be avoided and identity
preserved. In these examples each person could be described
as having demonstrated knowledge of their situation and
reflection on experiences. Reference to personal, familial
and social resources in order to bring the story to life for
the listener also appeared to be in evidence. Much has
been written about the use of positioning by others in their
relationships with people who have dementia; however,
positioning is also used by people with dementia to achieve
positive outcomes in the face of threats to identity. Thinking

about positioning as an aspect of resilience could facilitate a greater understanding as to how people with dementia respond to malignant positioning (Sabat, 2006) by others.

Loss of mastery and control, and loss of self-efficacy, are the associated risks in this theme, increasing the risk of low self-esteem. This can be seen where the person concerned appears to be defined by dementia. This doesn't mean hiding the fact that you are living with dementia, but rather, that there is a resignation by the person that their life is now limited by dementia. Sometimes this can be accepting the limitations that others place upon you which Kate Swaffer (2014) termed (and trademarked) as 'prescribed disengagement' following her own experiences of this. This is where the person concerned feels unable or unwilling to challenge misperceptions about them or their life with dementia or to stand up to infringements on their domestic citizenship in the home. This can also occur through contact with practitioners and support staff. Care and support can be stigmatising and can erode a person's sense of self. Helen, a social worker, picked this up in her work with Beth.

'I think some of the outcomes we talked about jointly together were about Beth maintaining her independence. She wanted to do that, and it was about finding ways for that to work for her. She needed more formal support to maintain friendships and make new friends and she decided to try day care. We also managed to support her with a personal support worker three times a week to meet her social needs. She needed practical help with housekeeping, shopping, budgeting. Day-to-day things. Well, there's levels and levels of dependence and independence. We were and are able to support Beth to be independent by offering appropriate help which she accepts to maximise her opportunities to be social on her own terms. But it is also about how help is given. You know she is worried about being considered round the twist or a charity case, as she calls it. She will be incredulous at times saying, "Why I am getting all this attention?" You know support is stigmatising.'

Meaning Making

Lots of people equate change, such as a declining memory, with just getting older. Hearing that you have dementia can then be a shock, resulting in a personal crisis, affecting every area of life. This can lead to feelings of shame, generalised anxiety, and even anticipatory mourning. Questions of, 'Am I still me?' or, 'Will I still be me tomorrow?' cause us to face an uncertain future, with this uncertainty experienced at the very core of our being. Resilience can be demonstrated where people can find a way to make sense of this new life. This is referred to as meaning making. Meaning making can occur in several ways: reflecting on the self over the life course, developing our own measure of what a good enough life looks like, and developing our own theories about why life turns out the way it does.

Reflections on Adversity across the Life Course

People with dementia reflect on difficult circumstances in their life. This can then serve as a comparison with the present problem or as a point of reference or reflection, and thus be used to gain insights into coping options within the current situation in which one finds oneself. This is part of the process of holding on to a sense of self as the person reflects on former coping mechanisms and tries to measure the present against these, or he or she attempts to employ these tried-and-tested coping mechanisms in the present.

Ellen describes her experiences as a carer for her husband, mother and children.

> 'Oh yes, I had no health problems or there was a sort of one point I got very depressed but, but then my mother she was living on her own and she became sort of, unwell she came here too, so, so! My husband eventually, the thing with him was that he was having falls he... I just couldn't cope with it. I couldn't lift him up... Anyway, I eventually got him into a nursing home. Well, the thing is you can't go, "Well, to hell with this" and just walk out... But there was a point when I felt very depressed and I was on anti-depressants. And then I had my mother come she had had a breakdown and the thing was I really couldn't go out and leave her with my toddlers. It wasn't that she would be violent but just things would go wrong... I, just didn't want to join in. I wasn't part of anything... I went into myself as it were. Because I really have no commitments now. If I had a lot or I couldn't do certain things or I wouldn't be able to leave family but I don't do a great deal now but I know I can do things if I want to.'

Ellen advises that she felt trapped by these responsibilities, resulting in an episode of depression. She uses narrative openness to share the realities of caring from her experience and the emotional impact of the situation. Ellen's story is an example of how the experience of adversity in the past can help build resilience in the present. Ellen uses her experiences to reflect on her life with dementia now and employs autobiographical reasoning to make comparisons. Ellen expresses a fear of losing her independence to others. Not having responsibilities and being able to go out as she pleases is an indicator of wellbeing for Ellen.

Alan uses autobiographical reasoning to reflect on his previous experiences of death and war. He recalls the personal and harrowing experience of being present when his father died suddenly.

'The night my father died I was at the house. What a night that was. He went to the toilet and I went behind him and he started being sick. I had to get a doctor out as soon as I could as he was coughing up blood. That lasted a few minutes and then he sort of went down on his knees and that was that. Well, I just had to deal with that as my mother was in the house, you know? It was an ordeal or an event that I will never forget, you know? Yes it was the worst thing that happened to me although during the war you know I saw some sights there. Some nights you would be going for your dinner and you would smell burning flesh if there had been a crash near the airfield but I coped then and I'm coping now. I have to, I have a wife... Well, it was frightening at first being away from home and doing a new job. I, I, I didn't know the area. It was in England but you soon adapt. Maybe that's why I mentioned it because we are talking about my attitude. It was a long time ago. Well, I was frightened. We all were. I didn't know what was going to happen to me. You lived every day as though it might be your last. I got up every morning scared about what might happen or what I might see but I still got up. But everyone did but we never mentioned how we felt. Well, everyone knew, because we all felt it...we just didn't say it... Well, you can't just sit about when there's a war on. I was needed to do a job I couldn't say I can't do that I have dementia? You always think about a war if you've experienced one.'

This was the worst thing to happen to Alan. He reminds himself that he survived this event and, therefore, can also survive with dementia. At the time of his father's death Alan prioritised the needs of his mother over and above his own grief. At this time he prioritises the needs of his wife over and above his own fears about dementia. Alan uses the phrase 'there's a war on' in the present tense within his story about living with dementia. His references to coping are about survival. He makes an association between being at war and having dementia. It is the story of the continuation of self in the face of dementia. The continual nature of *surviving* is conveyed in Alan's statement that every day could be your last.

In Ellen and Alan's stories they appear to use previous experiences and knowledge to assess threats to self in the present, with each person arriving at a different conclusion. Ellen is reassured; Alan is afraid. However, both appear to make the necessary adjustments through their personal resilience resources to live with dementia. What is interesting is that Ellen has taken comfort from being independent and having no responsibilities whilst Alan is reassured by his connections and responsibilities. This highlights the unique nature of each person's resilience and the dangers of generalising or making assumptions about vulnerability and protective factors.

Developing Your Own Measure of Good Enough

People with dementia often have their own ideas about how much being older and/or having dementia has had an impact on them. This involves elements of self-appraisal and testing the continuation of self. Setting criteria for personal decisions about 'doing okay' (Harris, 2008) and assessing self against these criteria reveals that memory, and the act of forgetting, can play a central role in the resilience of a person with dementia. However, it is not the ability to remember that appears important, rather, it is the person's own interpretation of how important the information was that has been forgotten. So, forgetting is not in itself a primary concern for people when assessing if they are 'good enough'. Instead, this is measured through a focus on living with memory loss; accepting that forgetting is now part of life; assuming anything that is forgotten is not important to begin with (even where others challenge you on this); a focus on wellbeing as an indicator of being healthy; and, finally, a sense of self as unchanged despite experiencing short-term memory loss. However, a note of caution: an insistence that you are doing okay despite evidence to the contrary could be evidence of the absence of personal adjustment strategies. In this case, such an insistence could be evidence of low resilience. I will return to this later in practice scenarios.

Making Sense: Personal Theories about Ageing and Dementia

Personal theories about your circumstances, including living with dementia, appear to have an important role in supporting a person's sense of self and status. Personal theories about ageing and/or dementia are important as they set the context for the master narrative of each person's story. Dora is a spiritual person and as a result uses her faith to both understand and cope with the changes in her health and her dementia.

'My memory is not so good so I can't remember exact dates or anything but I do know there came a time and I knew that that was the life for me and I gave my heart to the Lord and held him in it… Oh yes! He is with you.

The Lord doesn't say believe in me and I'll give you a good life. What he does is helps you through all of the bad things and it's a lifeline. He's there helping and you know you only need to turn to him and he will give you the grace to do something… I did go and see someone and told them what I did and they said, "You do the best thing you can do and you're doing it yourself, you're writing down important things." I wasn't worried about dementia or what they might tell me. I know what like I am in myself and I'm ready to meet the Lord and that was me. So I always know I was never alone even though there wasn't another human person here to speak to but I could speak to the Lord. That's what's brought me through everything!'

Spiritual or philosophical models of coming to terms with a health crisis, including dementia, can be an opportunity to gain insights into the self under pressure (Jacobson, 1993). Dora's religion is an important part of her identity and her motivation in life. As a result she contextualises her experience of adversity as a test from God. Dora believes that this is a test of her continued faith in the face of adversity. Within this, she balances her ill-health against the positives in her life, such as owning her home, a family who care for her, her love of the church and the opportunities she had to travel. Dora doesn't expect God to solve her problems but rather employs self-directed religious coping (Pargament *et al.*, 2000). This is where a person believes that God gives them the strength to deal with negative events and endure them with dignity. Dora states that God does not give you more than you can handle. This personal understanding means that Dora sees herself and her circumstances as significant, part of a bigger picture, and this gives her experience of dementia meaning and purpose.

Beth believes that dementia is her body's way of protecting her from terrible memories. She lost her son, Bobby, when he was a young man.

'Deaths in the family affected me awful bad. The death of anybody. Wee Bobby, wee Bobby. But what can a woman do? He was dead anyway. I can't really remember. I don't really know. Someone came up and told me what had happened. Aye, the police came up and told me. I can't really remember. The dementia. I don't want to remember. Aye, aye, I don't want to remember and my body knows that… I think if I remember. I think that something bad happened and because of that my memory just went [*makes a whistling noise and uses hand to indicate going over her head*]. My body just wanted me to forget it. You know? I think, aye, I think it's something like that. But if I really want to remember something I have to write it down. I don't want to think about it. My memory is bad because of this terrible thing, you know? My body doesn't want to remember. And I'm very happy really. I'm very happy here.'

Beth focuses on the positive impact of memory loss. She believes that her body 'created dementia' to facilitate a sense of peace or respite from painful memories. Dementia is re-framed by Beth as a means of 'pain management' from upsetting memories and emotions. She is then able to focus on the positive things in her life. This personal theory positions Beth in a survivor discourse, where she is surviving the emotional pain of her previous trauma. This approach could also be an example of intersectional reserve (Hulko, 2009). Beth has had to endure many difficult experiences in her life. It is possible that in the context of such experiences memory loss, as a result of dementia, may be just one more thing to contend with, and not really of that much significance in the grand scheme of a person's life. This can be surprising to practitioners who often believe that dementia is experienced as devastating to the person. Beth's story demonstrates that this isn't always the case.

Personal theories appear to be an essential part of the continual process of adjustment. They provide a context for each person to manage day-to-day experiences of ageing, ill-health or dementia. The accuracy of each person's theory does not seem to have any bearing on effectiveness. What appears to be important is the investment that the person has in these theories. The stories that the person tells then work towards supporting these personal understandings, and, in turn, they preserve our sense of self. However, it can also be argued that fixed personal theories can be used to deny threats and problems. It is, therefore, important within a resilience context to be able to differentiate between those personal theories that support adjustments, and those which might make adaptation less likely. For example, 'there is nothing wrong'. Ignoring a situation will never resolve it. This includes the subject of dementia. Therefore, an absence of meaning making or little opportunity for meaning making is the third risk category. This is sometimes referred to as a 'lack of insight' where the person concerned denies that they have dementia or that they are experiencing any problems. An insistence that you are 'doing okay' despite evidence to the contrary would also be an example.

Where does this take us? Well, this more detailed exploration of the responses of people with dementia brings to life the quiet, active nature of resilience. This facilitates a more sensitive approach to revealing the protective and risk factors for each person. The Risk and Protective Factors Quick Rating Tool (Table 5.1) is a handy way to focus on the areas that need more support. We can then refer back to the Resilience Reserve in order to find resources to enhance protective factors and decrease risks, or to identify gaps where we might need to assist.

Table 5.1 Risk and Protective Factors Quick Rating Tool

Protective Factors	Score Protective Factors 1–5 Strongly Agree 5 Agree 4 Mostly Agree 3 Disagree 2 Strongly Disagree 1	Risk Factors
Sense of being connected to people and places *Comments:*	Rewarding relationships with others *Score:* Sense of belonging *Score:* I still feel like me *Score:*	Isolation/ disconnectedness *Comments:*
Sense of mastery and control, self-efficacy and self-esteem *Comments:*	Feels able to influence events and people in his or her life *Score:* Is confident in self if a problem arises *Score:* Feels good about self or achievements in life *Score:*	Loss of mastery and control, self-efficacy, self-esteem *Comments:*
Meaning making *Comments:*	I feel that I am doing okay *Score:* My life makes sense to me *Score:*	No meaning making/ lack of opportunity for meaning making *Comments:*

The quick rating scale is based on the relationship between protective and risk factors, for example having a sense of connectedness versus feelings of disconnectedness. By asking questions about protective factors we can, therefore also highlight risks and vulnerabilities.

Being able to sensitively appraise these factors is, however, dependent on spending time getting to know the person, and hearing their stories. Assessment is one of the ways in which we do this in work with people living with dementia. The next chapter will explore this in more detail.

CHAPTER 6

Locating Resilience in Everyday Stories

Before we begin, let us recap on what we have discussed so far. Resilience is developed in the face of adversity. The experience of dementia can be understood as one of adversity, holding on to a sense of self in the face of threats to identity. It is, therefore, possible for resilience to emerge in the experience of dementia. The presence of resilience doesn't mean that the person does not experience the emotional impact of dementia, such as grief, loss or anxiety, or fears about what the future might hold. However, it does lessen the impact of these and facilitates adaptation to events despite this, through the mobilisation and employment of assets and resources. So, living with dementia, whatever that might mean for that person within the context of their own life, involves continual responses to both small and larger changes and new experiences. The shifting sands of dementia can make any sense of continuity, and in turn security, difficult to achieve. The assets and resources that we have in our personal toolkit are, therefore, extremely important. When a person has dementia they might forget about long-standing skills or lose confidence in their ability to respond as a result of the label 'dementia'. And so, help is needed to visualise the assets and resources at hand. These resources then have to be employed, at the right time, for the right effect. Again, assistance might be required to do this. What is clear is that in order to assist the person concerned, practitioners need to listen carefully to understand each person, and bring to life this Resilience Reserve. Assessment is a key component of how we learn about others, and so we will now turn our attention to this.

Assessment holds the key to gathering all of the information we need. But what do we mean by assessment? Essentially, we want to know the person better. Who is this person and what matters to them? What are the things that are important to them and their wellbeing? However, rather than being seen as a tool for inquiry and a means of finding out more about someone, assessments are often, instead, viewed as necessary organisational paperwork. Because assessment is so closely aligned with resource allocation it can often be approached as a checklist focusing on need and risk. The bureaucratic function of the document can then be prioritised over its analytical role in our work. As a result there can be a tendency to focus on 'what's wrong with you?' Why is this important? Opportunities to reveal resilience sit within the broader framework of interpretation or finding meaning. Assessment is the application of theoretical, personal and procedural knowledge in a situation to determine meaning. This is what we call the *assessment process*. We can then produce a written assessment record with the purpose of care planning (O'Connor *et al.*, 2006).

In addition, people with dementia can also find that they have a lesser role in assessment interactions. How often do we prioritise the accounts of other people, for example, family members, rather than really focusing on what the subject of the assessment, that is the person with dementia, is trying to convey? In 2014, researchers Österholm and Samuelsson analysed interactions in five assessment meetings between social workers and a person with dementia. In each of these assessment meetings a family member or friend was also in attendance. They identified several phenomena taking place in these meetings that worked to position the person with dementia as less competent than the person without dementia. This included the social worker ignoring the person with dementia and focusing on the answers and views of the family member; posing questions that implied a lack of competence on behalf of the person with dementia; using phrases, such as 'we' as in 'we think that's best', which implied that prior discussions and decisions had already been made, and using the person's first name routinely without checking that it was appropriate to do so. So, assessments are not neutral tools that reflect a single truth; instead, they reflect the position, values and focus of the practitioner who is undertaking the assessment. We need to think more creatively about assessment and the tools that we use when a person has dementia. This includes an emphasis on stories to reveal the personal nature of threats and the ways in which people respond. Assessments used correctly can also provide creative ways of recording individual, community and organisational assets, as well as highlighting the things that might be missing, and, thus, provide a focus for intervention.

The Importance of Everyday Stories of Life with Dementia

Approaching assessment from a narrative or storytelling perspective provides a vehicle to avoid or address negatively positioning a person living with dementia. It does this by generating a co-constructed meaning of 'this life with dementia'. Such approaches are still relatively rare. The stories we tell about ourselves and our lives are socially and culturally located, and as such their inclusion and analysis in assessment practice is relevant and valid. In this way, assessments can reveal the citizenship of people living with dementia. There can, however, be practical difficulties in hearing the stories of people with dementia. We often listen for chronological or logical connections in narratives. As a result stories that are considered illogical or confused are often dismissed or used as evidence of cognitive decline within assessments (Young, 2010). However, all stories have the potential to reveal important information about character, themes and personal values. Stories can often offer insights into a person's sense of self at the point of the interaction. This provides opportunities for unique outcomes and personal solutions to the issues that people face, with the opportunity for more effective, meaningful engagement in people's lives as we discover important relationships and attachments and uncover stories of resilience and survival. We also know that the content of a person's thoughts are conveyed to others through words and actions, including behaviour and non-verbal communication. Even when the wrong words are used, gestures, tone of voice and expression can convey what a person is thinking and feeling. All of us who work with people with dementia can, therefore, engage with the individual using stories to explore and validate resilient identities in hidden discourse. The better we know the person the easier this is to achieve.

Everyday Magic (My Interpretation of Masten's Ordinary Magic)

Stories and conversations help us to understand the complex interaction of vulnerability and protective factors that are at play within the context of adversity and resilience. They do this by providing the context for these interacting factors. We can then learn from these stories about the person's feelings, opinions and motivations, as they describe events within these accounts. My own research was undertaken using this narrative approach that can be replicated in care and practice situations. This involves finding a way to facilitate the person concerned leading on topics, and taking the conversation in different directions, which is sometimes confusing for the listener. At other times, prompts might be needed to encourage this free-flowing approach. Then, using thematic analysis (looking for story themes) I deconstructed the stories into smaller stories. I explored what each story revealed about this person, their associated feelings, attitudes, actions and motivations. I also considered which stories appeared to have particular importance to the individual as well as noting the other people (characters) who featured, and the ways in which the person with dementia chose to portray themselves. In essence, what did this person want me to know about him or her, the people in their life and what had happened? An open narrative approach to assessment encourages stories and storytelling; a reflective approach of listening to understand and not simply to reply or assert your own views as 'expert'; and for the listener to clarify where questions are needed. This encourages a dynamic experience for both the person with dementia and the practitioner and is displayed in Figure 6.1.

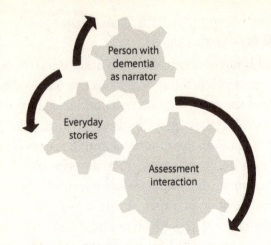

Figure 6.1 The Dynamic Narrative Assessment Process

A Dynamic, Respectful Assessment Process

A dynamic, narrative assessment process can be criticised for being too unstructured by some, whereas the opposite may be the case. Such an approach is structured by the narrator, in this case the person living with dementia. The listener (the practitioner) can ask questions, informed by theory and practice knowledge, in order to delve further into stories or to encourage stories about specific areas of a person's life. The important thing is to allow the person to set the pace and not to dismiss stories that appear off topic or irrelevant. It is often the conversations shared before the assessment 'interview' begins that can be the most important. Planning for the assessment must be done with care and includes maximising the personal control of the narrator, and ensuring the person with dementia is enabled to participate in their own time and at their own pace. This means we are creating a shared space built on equity between listener and narrator. We do this by:

- enabling choice

- respecting humanness and personal dignity

- preserving continuity for the person with
  dementia (Cox *et al.*, 1998, p.23).

People with dementia have varying experiences of dementia and different degrees of cognitive impairment. It is, therefore, essential to build time into the assessment interaction process. Communicating with people who live with dementia is about communicating on their terms. This was confirmed by the Scottish Dementia Working Group, Research Sub-Group in their 2014 paper on this subject which referred to this as respecting 'dementia time' (p.684). It involves respecting each person's abilities and reality, not imposing our reality and time pressures into the interaction. The more pressured an interaction is, in terms of time or information demands, the less equitable the space we share becomes. So, simply, create space, time and calm, to let the person tell their own story.

Set the Scene for a Good Story

The environment also plays a pivotal role in either enhancing or detracting from effective communication. The place in which the assessment takes place should be somewhere familiar to the person concerned. Many people with dementia experience sensory challenges alongside the other changes associated with dementia (Houston and Christie, 2018). This can mean that the person has problems with vision, hearing or acoustic sensitivity and perception, to name but a few. Before beginning you should ensure that the environment is quiet with no distractions, and that the person with dementia is able to hear and understand you, and see your face. Every care must be taken in narrative work. The lived experience of telling one's story can be upsetting and be the source of possible distress. Good practice is dependent on self-regulation by the listener in judging the mood of the participant and stopping the assessment interaction where this is required. People we work with are not under any obligation to discuss any issues that they do not wish to disclose and can stop interactions at any point. Time must also be built into the process to respond to emotional disclosures and possible upset. In this respect the listener is accountable to the person. This accountability is further demonstrated through ensuring that each person has choice over the preferred venue, duration and times of the scheduled meetings and the presence of others. This is of particular importance due to the effects of tiredness on cognition (Robinson, 2002).

What happens when despite this the assessment narrative is still mixed up, or the person has problems communicating, or the story doesn't seem to make chronological sense? Is it even factually correct? This is when we can use storyboards.

Storyboards

Storyboards are traditionally used to plot storytelling in film. Using a combination of images and words, storyboards facilitate an impression of the story which is envisioned long before the completed whole (Sova and Sova, 2006). You can use this approach to build a single visual structure of the emerging story. You start with a blank canvas which names the person and their story, and then identify the key opening and closing story points of the master narrative. From here you then add the details of the smaller stories, and use the storyboard template to place these within the larger story, to gain a sense of the overall story trajectory (see Table 6.1).

Below each of these smaller stories you can add layers of story content. This allows you to see a whole story and story process for each person. A storyboard offers a flexible way of creating levels of understanding so that you can quickly see how many small stories make the building bricks of the larger ones. Stories are revealed as multi-layered and story trajectories become visible. New possibilities are revealed between the content and the potential purpose of each narrative. This approach enables us to keep the whole story in mind, whilst at the same time paying due attention to seemingly insignificant content. This is a great way to reveal the subtle threats experienced by a person which aren't always expressly stated. It is this analytical exploration of everyday stories which sets them apart from a conversation. Table 6.1 is a storyboard template that can be used if you want to try this approach. You can populate the table with words, images and photos.

Table 6.1 Storyboard Template

	Storyboard
Story title	
Plotline (what is this story about?)	
Characters (who is in the story?)	
Outcome (what happens?)	
Purpose (what does the person want me to know?)	
Meaning (what is this story really about?)	
Identity/sense of self (how does the story teller want me to see him or her?)	

When I have used this approach I have been struck by the depth of the stories shared by the person with dementia. It is humbling to be trusted with the intimate nature of another's stories about self, society and observations on life. The stories told by people with dementia can be dismissed as non-factual or superficial, assumed to have no substance or purpose. However, I have found that the stories told by people with dementia can, in fact, be rich repositories of information. In particular, stories can reveal insights into what might constitute a better than expected outcome for that particular individual, and without that story, these important aspects of life can remain hidden from view. They are, therefore, powerful and at the same time sensitive and must be treated with respect. This applies to the act of generating stories together, but also in handling stories as they are transformed into narratives for assessment processes and analysis. Stories offer points of reflection and re-positioning for the people that we work with. The active nature of these aspects of story reveal the ways in which people with dementia can possibly regain power within interactions. The act of storytelling in and of itself, therefore, provides an opportunity for resilience to be realised. Invitations to tell the story of self can, in their own right, be a catalyst for resilience to be realised, in that moment, for people with dementia. I have found that the use of storyboards is not well known or used within practice situations. They are, however, a very accessible practice tool with which to engage with theories, knowledge and evidence practically as part of the assessment process. Surface stories can be built upon and critically analysed through the application of theory, knowledge, skills and values. Additional layers which represent associated policy and legislation can also be applied. My experience of using storyboards has led me to believe that this is an under-used resource in practice and in the communication of our practice with others, offering a perspective on the processes at play.

The purpose of this book is to consider how we can take a concept like resilience and apply it to real experiences of living with dementia, caring for a person with dementia and practice with people living with dementia. So far, we have discussed the threats and the impact of threats through an exploration of protective and risk factors. We will now focus on the Resilience Reserve and the ways in which we can visualise each person's assets and resources in order to mobilise these and support areas where there may be a gap or vulnerability. A suggested template is given in Table 6.2. We need to be mindful that the domains are interconnected and must be considered as contextual. This personal Resilience Reserve is our bank of skills, experiences and knowledge, including personal, familial, social, financial and political resources which we build over our lifetime. It is our Resilience Reserve that we each refer to in order to enact our problem-solving solutions.

In order to do this, we need to recognise our individual, community and organisational assets, and have the ability to mobilise and utilise these to where they are needed and to when they are needed. A robust reserve ensures that we are able to successfully resolve issues and builds self-confidence. This trust in ourselves, as someone who can cope, becomes part of our persona and forms the building blocks of our continued resilience. For people living with dementia, help can be needed to hold on to this self-knowledge. Other people can misinterpret the responses of the person, and opportunities to problem solve can be missed. This can then have the opposite effect of losing confidence in self and becoming disempowered as others find solutions for us, or our solutions are not valued. Practically, a resilience framework is a useful way to approach support planning with a person with dementia and their family. The support and wellbeing of carers is also an essential part of the equation. You can use the Resilience Reserve model in work with carers, as well as work with the person with dementia, and indeed, in doing so, it provides an opportunity to compare factors within caring and interdependent dyads. It provides an opportunity to look at the pooled resources within care partnerships. Where resources can be shared, this model provides an opportunity to use resilience to further strengthen the shared experience of finding ways to cope. Where there are differences, this model can help carers gain an insight into why the person with dementia is responding in the way they are. An example of working with the model in this way is presented in Chapter 8.

This approach is compatible with citizenship and human rights focused practice. Re-framing all of our lives as interconnected and seeing each other as interdependent citizens could be a useful approach. It also opens up opportunities for support relationships to be defined by those involved, rather than simply referring to 'the dependent person with dementia' and 'their carer'. Instead, both parties can be considered as contributing in different ways within interdependent relationships. Opportunities to realise resilience could then be promoted. There are some prompt questions (see Table 6.2) to help populate this content but it is not an exhaustive list and you may find you have other questions and insights as you talk to people. You can also use this scale personally as well as completing it for other people. In addition to showing the range of resources that you have access to, you can also use this approach to see those domains that are not as robust as others and that need to be supported.

Table 6.2 Resilience Domain Topics

Domains	Content Topics	Content Notes
Experiences	What I want you to know about me	
	Key points in my life – chronology	
	Stories of interest	
	Education/life events/ work	
	What is happening now?	
	How I feel and why	
	My care and support needs	
Roles	My relationships	
	People who depend on me	
	How I make myself available to others	
	Work and community roles	
	Spiritual and cultural roles	
	Who would be impacted if I wasn't there?	
Knowledge, Skills and Interests	The things I am good at (my talents)	
	What I can do	
	Hobbies and interests (what I like to do)	
	What I have learned and what I know	
	I can apply what I know to different situations	

Domains	Content Topics	Content Notes
Personal Qualities	What I want other people to say about me/how I want to be known	
	What other people would say about me	
	What I like about myself	
	What type of person I am	
	Things I would change about myself	
Assets and Resources	The people, places and things that are important to me/that I rely on and value	
	The place where I live	
	The person who knows me best	
	Friends	
	Pets	
	My community and neighbourhood	
	My home and the things I own	
	My financial situation	
	Getting about/transport links	
	Sources of help or assistance	
	People I can turn to	
	Care and support that I receive	
	What I have to offer	
	Someone to talk to	

Motivation	What I want to do and why	
	What is important to me	
	What I would like to happen now	
	Personal theories about my life	

A Resilience-Focused Example

Michael works in a care home. He is the key worker for a group of residents, one of whom is Noreen. Noreen has recently been diagnosed with Alzheimer's disease. She was a district nurse before she retired, and moved into residential care five years ago when her mobility had been affected by arthritis. Over the past year she has been increasingly forgetful and anxious. Recently, she forgot the name of her grandson when he visited and this greatly upset her. Michael has spent a lot of time with Noreen. He knows how important her family life is to her. Michael began by using a narrative approach to listen carefully to Noreen. Noreen was potentially at risk from becoming disconnected from her family. She had asked her daughter not to visit because she was now anxious ahead of planned visits. Michael is concerned that Noreen is at risk of isolation as she tries to avoid this situation happening again. He has also found written notes with family names crumpled up in the pockets of Noreen's clothes. He wonders if this is an attempt by Noreen to gain some control over her memory loss. He wants to help Noreen find a way to manage this without causing her anxiety or losing valuable time with her family. Using the Quick Rating Tool (Table 5.1) Michael summarises the issues (Table 6.3).

Table 6.3 Michael's Notes (1)

Protective Factors	Score Protective Factors 1–5 Strongly Agree 5 Agree 4 Mostly Agree 3 Disagree 2 Strongly Disagree 1	Risk Factors
Sense of connection to people and places *Comments: Family visit regularly. She is at home here and is happy. This new problem of forgetting family has thrown her.*	Rewarding relationships with others *Score: 2* Sense of belonging *Score:4* I still feel like me *Score: 2*	Isolation/ disconnectedness *Comments: Noreen doesn't want her family to visit due to her memory worries. She isn't enjoying her time with them because of this and is upset when they leave.*
Sense of mastery and control, self-efficacy and self-esteem *Comments: Noreen hasn't been able to find a solution to this problem and is uncertain about what this means.*	Feels able to influence events and people in his or her life *Score: 2* Is confident in self if a problem arises *Score: 2* Feels good about self or achievements in life *Score: 3*	Loss of Mastery and Control, self-efficacy, self-esteem *Comments: Noreen's self-esteem has been affected by this issue. She feels she is losing control to dementia.*
Meaning making	I feel that I am doing okay *Score: 2* My life makes sense to me *Score: 3*	No meaning making/ lack of opportunity for meaning making *Comments: Noreen can't understand why this is happening.*

He then refers to the Resilience Reserve domains to build a picture of the assets and resources that Noreen might have access to, in order to reduce risk factors and promote the protective factors. An extract from Michael's notes are as follows (Table 6.4):

Table 6.4 Michael's Notes (2)

Noreen's Unique Resilience Reserve	Michael's Notes
Motivation	To continue to be an active member of the family and to be thought of as 'present' in the company of others.
Experiences	Previous experience of coping with adversity. Strong female role models. Supporting others in need. Happy family life.
Roles	Nurse Mother Grandmother Wife Neighbour
Knowledge and skills	Good listener/communication skills Organisational skills Approachable Good education Supporting others Articulate Knowledge of adversity in other people's lives through nursing

Michael decides to approach the topic by reminding Noreen of the importance of family in her life. Together they then explore the concerns she has about what could happen during a visit and how this would make her feel. Noreen is worried about what forgetting family means, but also about how she would appear in the eyes of her family as a diminished or changed version of herself. Noreen and Michael create a visual representation of the Resilience Reserve domains, using photos and notes. Michael notes that during this activity Noreen focuses on her work as a nurse. She marvels at how she had managed to remember lots of information. But as she and Michael discuss this, they begin to reveal the different tools Noreen had used to manage her work. They then dig deeper into the Resilience Reserve by focusing on the role of *nurse* and drilling down into the knowledge, skills and interests that Noreen had used to manage her work-related tasks to see if any of these could work for her now. These are listed in Table 6.5.

Table 6.5 Michael's Notes (3)

Noreen's Knowledge, Skills and Experiences	Michael's Notes
Nurse – managing work-related demands	Working with others in a team. Daily report of tasks to be completed. Diary of meetings and who would be there. Debrief with team members.

Michael and Noreen look at this list of Noreen's work management routine in the context of her memory loss worries. This is the plan they develop. They begin by identifying who Noreen's 'team' would be to help her with this issue. This consists of Michael and two members of the care team. In the morning someone will check in with Noreen and provide her with a 'report' of what is to come that day, including planned family visits. They also check this against her diary to ensure all the details needed are there. Noreen also keeps her diary with notes with her, and has her diary open during her family's visits so that she can refer to it. After each visit Noreen speaks to a member of her 'team' to discuss any changes that might be needed in her diary notes ahead of the next visit. They also keep the option open of including Noreen's daughter in the 'support team' when Noreen feels that she can be more open about her fears in this area with her family.

Prioritising the Everyday

What does this focus on resilience-based solutions allow us to do? Dealing with forgetfulness and maintaining relationships in dementia care isn't really seen as a priority. These activities are often seen by organisations as of a low priority with support geared towards personal care and avoiding risks, essentially turning the conversation from one of 'need for support' to 'need for resource'. The valuable contribution that support workers make through the type of support provided by Michael, for example, can make all the difference. Our care tasks can be viewed as a series of isolated activities. Resilience is a way of making visible how they, in fact, contribute to the whole person and their continued sense of self, promoting resilience, and in turn, more rewarding practice for those engaged in this work. This approach to care and support is person centred, asset based and employs co-production. This is also a good example of how something that can be seen as 'normal' or expected when a person has dementia, such as memory loss, can have a profound impact on a person's sense of self.

Helping people to compensate through their own skill reserves can go a long way to promoting resilience. The key points are that we:

- reduce stressors

- facilitate time and space for the person to function at their best

123

- improve the environment by providing cues

- improve communication

- build continuity into everything we do

- be flexible and authentic in our approach

- see people as individuals and develop individual strategies

- support carers and others in the person's network

- provide the right resources at the right time

- ask what can you do; what can I do; and what can we do?

'Person in situation'

The phrase 'person in situation' was first used by Coulshed and Orme (1998, p.134) to describe psycho-social approaches to social work practice. I have used 'person in situation' to describe a particular approach where a person's assessment story is contextualised and reflects his or her life view. The person is portrayed as an active participant. The story is from their own perspective. This facilitates an interpretation of events and circumstances. We can do this through simple things, such as not referring to the people we work with as clients or residents, but instead using a preferred name. Using resilience in practice is a 'person in situation' approach that requires time, sensitivity and respect. It keeps the person at the centre of support planning by consistently contextualising issues and problems from his or her perspective. This approach respects the everyday rituals that make up a person's life and provide meaning. It then uses a co-production approach to problem solve without rushing to traditional service responses. It creates a space for creativity and more rewarding relationships between people living with dementia and the people who support them. However, practitioners who want to work in this way can experience tensions as a result of the expectations of others, including their organisations. The next chapter will explore this in more detail.

CHAPTER 7

Practice Tensions in the Search for Resilience

Organisational identity and the influence of organisations, politics and policy can complicate attempts to find resilience in our work with people living with dementia. Although not everyone living with dementia can be resilient, the possibility of resilience exists despite dementia. However, unless this possibility of resilience is facilitated by practitioners it may never be realised. Competing demands between the way that we would like to work, the resources available to us in our work, and the demands of our organisations can stop us working in the way that we would aspire to. Risk is closely associated with people with dementia generally. As a result, practice with people with dementia can very easily become risk-focused and not person-focused. The expectations and needs of other people, within the person's care and support network, can also be prioritised over and above the needs of the person living with dementia. All of this means that human service professionals can experience tensions between practice, roles and values as we try to achieve the best for the people that we work with.

Competing Demands
Organisational Identity Versus Our Sense of Self

Working in care and support is hard. Tensions can occur when competing priorities are in evidence. For example, practitioners may be viewed as the experts or 'problem solvers' when they begin to work with families. However, practitioners are often not in positions of autonomy, and have to negotiate organisational gatekeeping to access resources, and have care plans approved. An emphasis on organisational objectives and process can minimise the opportunities to identify and promote resilience in people with dementia.

Gwen is a social worker who works with older people in a local authority social work team. She has recently completed an assessment of need for a man living with dementia. Gwen explains that an emphasis on need is a requirement to acquire support for people.

'I am very aware that you need to see people over two or three visits, so they don't tire as well. But you also want to get the services they need in as soon as you can. So it's a constant challenge. I feel under pressure to get the information quickly and generate a paper assessment, but the process of writing is also a reflective exercise where you can re-visit what you've been told and think about the emphasis that the person placed on seemingly mundane information. I identified that he needed total assistance with some personal care and prompting and guidance in other areas. His wife did need to know support was available as she was exhausted. This sounds terrible but, and I don't just mean for my client, you are making the person sound not as good as they are. You don't promote their strengths or you won't get resources. What I mean is you emphasise the things the person can't do and play down the writing around strengths. I'm not making anything up about him but I am emphasising the things I know will secure me resources.'

This approach prevents resilience being realised. At worst it perpetuates the social frame of the 'vulnerable person with dementia in need' in both written and verbal assessments. The result of this is that the person can never be realised as a citizen with the capacity for resilience. This influences the positions that we take in our practice and the ways in which we position the people with dementia that we work with. The tensions caused by the competing demands of organisational processes and priorities, and the individual values and practice approaches that practitioners strive to implement, are central to changing how we see people who need support, and the type of support that we prioritise. It is important to acknowledge these tensions as the context within which practice with people ageing with dementia takes place. This provides important detail as to the context within which both citizenship and resilience are ignored or promoted. Compare this to Helen, who explicitly links characteristics, roles and experiences to the process of resilience and provides detailed information about the person she is working with, their life, the challenges that they have faced and their responses.

'She [Beth] appeared to be a very independent woman, who knows her own mind, who could state her case, enjoyed the fact that she saw herself as quite a tough cookie who could deal with things. Didn't really need other people's help… Well, she has a great sense of humour, she's a great laugh. She's a very hard-working woman. Has been all her days. Parents' deaths were difficult and the death of her grandmother hit her hard…

She had a very difficult marriage and she's happy to talk about these things openly. She wants to impress upon you that she's had difficulties in her life but she's coping. She's come out the other end and that's all part of her resilience. These traumatic incidents have, she advises, made her very strong and I would agree with that. Well, all these things could have broken other people… She has had huge upset and trauma in her family life and she talks about it openly. Her family is very important to her and she's worked very, very hard to bring her kids up and do her best by them. She had an abusive husband and she had to leave him and take the kids to stay with a friend and start all over again. So she's had huge crosses to bear… Beth has her inner strengths and qualities, she has a strong character and personality and most of those things have remained intact.'

This account facilitates a direct link for the listener between Beth the person, and Beth's skills, experiences, roles, resources, and resilience. Helen discusses the adversities Beth faced within the context of her relationships with others. Although Beth had experienced traumas, Helen does not define her by this. Instead, Helen focuses on aspects of Beth's identity that help her cope, and how Beth has become stronger through adversity. This would appear to be an example of Helen recognising the value of Beth's intersectional experiences, that is, the experience of divorce, hardship and coping with abuse, and the role that these can play in helping people to adjust to the changes that dementia can bring as described earlier in Chapter 2 (Hulko, 2009). This way of talking about the people that we work with reflects a narrative approach where the person with dementia is at the centre of their own story. Adversities that the person has experienced over their life are discussed, as well as the ways in which skills, experiences and resources contribute to adjustments to different circumstances throughout life. There are reflections on the person's sense of self and their public identity, how they are seen by service providers and practitioners, and the assumptions this leads to, which can bleed into practice and practice decisions. This is especially visible in discussions on risk.

Living with Risk

Barry (2007) stated that the literature on community care is highly critical of the emphasis on risk over and above care and treatment models, and recommends policy and practice initiatives that demonstrate confidence and commitment to encouraging people, rather than restricting capacities. Robinson *et al.* (2007) compared the views of people with dementia and professionals regarding risk. They found that professionals focus on the physical domain of risk such as harm, whereas people with dementia focus on the biographical domain such as loss of identity (p.401). Clarke *et al.* (2010) interviewed 55 people with dementia, carers and practitioners in order to identify contested areas of risk perspective. They identified these as: friendships, smoking, going out, domestic arrangements, occupation and activity. The authors concluded that continuing to engage in such activities was important for the identity of the person concerned. This opens up a new perspective on risk management as a building block in the continuity of self, placing practitioners at the heart of this through their practice relationships and responsibilities. Clarke and Bailey (2016, p.436) stated that more needs to be known about how people living with dementia, and the significant people in their lives, define and manage risk, and how they then draw on their own resilience to foster a sense of wellbeing, and achieve a good quality of life.

McDonald *et al.* (2008) identified three different roles adopted by social workers when working with people with dementia, described as legal representatives, protectors and advocates (pp.32–34). Legal representatives are positivist practitioners who seek structure, routine and prescribed responses to issues that arise. Protectors view those who lack capacity as unable to foresee and take precaution against obvious risks. They seek to persuade people with dementia to accept less risk associated activities. The third role of advocate is described as being explicitly person centred. Advocates have an acute awareness of the social construction of the identity *person with dementia* which results in a risk enablement approach, such as that promoted through the findings of Clarke *et al.* (2010). Manthorpe (2004, p.142) also explored this issue explicitly linking risk-averse practice and dementia to a wider discourse of ageism and oppression. To consider risk enablement and resilience as possibilities for people with dementia is to openly challenge these powerful constructs. Manthorpe cautioned that if people with dementia are seen as 'personifications of risk then there is a greater likelihood that fear and ignorance will govern assessment and risk management' (2004, p.148). This is similar to the themes raised by Bailey *et al.* (2013) in which people with dementia are inherently viewed as risky people. The roles adopted by practitioners in their work with a person with dementia have a direct impact on practice and outcomes. One of the reasons for this is the dichotomy between generalising about 'people with dementia' and seeing the individual living with dementia.

Person with Dementia Versus People with Dementia

Practitioners can find it difficult to differentiate between the homogeneous group 'people with dementia' and the individuality of the 'person with dementia'. As such, they can find it difficult to use resilience-based frameworks when they apply generalised understandings of dementia in their practice. Practitioners have to be aware of these generalised frames creeping into their practice unchallenged. In some cases, they can be examples of epistemic injustice as described by Young *et al.* (2019) who explained that assumptions about 'people' with dementia based on stereotypes can lead to prejudicial treatment of an individual with dementia. So, for example, 'people with dementia wander', therefore, 'this person with dementia will wander'. Practice then discriminates against the individual in the form of either 'I must restrict this person's movements or liberty' without engaging and hearing the person's individual story, or hearing the person but discounting what they have to say as you don't believe them to be a credible informer. Such frames of reference focus on risk and issues of safety over and above citizenship and human rights perspectives and make opportunities for resilience less visible. This can be recognised in two ways. The first is where people are discussed generically with reference to 'what people with dementia do'. The second is where a specific person with dementia is referred to. As a result, a different picture often emerges where the person is described as an individual who has life experiences and access to resources that can be employed in their day-to-day lives. Both of these approaches can be used at the same time and this reveals the competing nature of such frames and their influence on how we practise.

In this example, Doug, who is a social worker, emphasises the short-term memory loss and *frailty* of the person he is working with. He translates this into categories of risk and, in particular, the risk of falls and risk of going out alone.

'So her short-term memory was very poor. So that stuck out for me. I thought she has very poor short-term memory and she was frail and a high risk of falls. She had a community alarm in and I asked whether she was going out of her house and things like that, you know the more serious risks for people with dementia "Are they going out of their house?" and things like that and, touch wood, she hasn't and I don't think she ever will do anything like that. There's a sign on the door that says "please do not go out" and certainly I don't think she is ever going to do this… Her memory is the number one thing that is very much impaired and her cognitive ability is such that she can't carry out certain tasks but in terms of where she is and keeping safe she's got that ability. In that initial visit I didn't know that and when I saw that her memory was very poor and when I saw the note on the door I did ask, but knowing her now I know she wouldn't do that.'

Doug stresses that for people with dementia, the risk of 'them' going out is a major safety concern. He refers to the individuality of the specific person he is working with. However, the care planning focuses on avoiding activities and there is little discussion about the importance of staying connected or support to socialise. Instead, the person concerned has to reassure the social worker that she will stay in the house and Doug adopts the role of 'protector' (Barry, 2007).

This example from Helen, who works in a hospital team, contains a detailed exploration and rejection of generic understandings of dementia. Helen discusses how people with dementia can be defined by the help they need or the services that support them. Such approaches can de-personalise the individual concerned. Instead, Helen focuses on how assessments can be used to engage and see the person as an individual.

'For me…it's about not how somebody is functioning just now but it's about their history, who they were, and painting that picture and finding out about who they were, and how they functioned and what they did in their life and what their interests were. I think this is really important because what are assessments used for? Often in our business it's about providing information to other service providers so that they can work with the person. So it's important that they see that person and not just as "that's a tuck call" [a tuck call is local shorthand for a home care service to assist a person to bed] or that's "day care two days a week". To actually see the person so I provide points of reference in their personal history so that others can link in and engage with… It's about helping people to maintain the skills they already have and supporting them to come to terms with skills they have lost either emotionally or through practical support. It's about working with the person to fill some of these gaps and maintain a preferred way of life. Now some people want to be looked after and that's fine – it's not about what I think is good for someone. It's about helping people find the path for their life. Now the problem with dementia is that this isn't always clear or there might be difficulty understanding what a person feels or want. But through use of self, spending time, respecting a person's need for time and space and also privacy…but we have to also keep them safe and independent. Well is not just the bread and butter things like home care. I think social life is very important and engagement with the wider world, continued opportunities if you like.'

Dependent Independence

According to the Oxford dictionary, independence, or the state of being independent, is where *one is free from outside control and not subject to another's authority*. However, the word 'independence' is used in lots of ways in work with people with dementia. It can be used to describe an aspiration of the practitioner for the person that they are working with, and this is very relevant to re-ablement and rehabilitation discussions; as an indicator of how well the person is coping with life with dementia; as an indicator of how much support is required; and as a stated outcome of our interventions. It is frequently used in situations that imply outside influence on the person and/or the actions undertaken. In essence, this is a *dependent independence*. The phrase 'supported independence' (Hale *et al.*, 2010, p.2) has been used to denote the specific care work or support services that enable older people to continue to live at home. Hale *et al.* (p.2) suggested that independence is achieved through the control and autonomy that an older person can exert over the support they receive. However, this isn't the case for lots of people who live with dementia. Independence is discussed as a status that is granted by others and, more importantly, that can be removed by others. This is illustrated by Kate who works in a mental health team.

'I think like that initially I'm not challenging her views or anything and trying to explain if there is a difference between parties that we are just trying to help and just saying, "We are here to help." And she doesn't really acknowledge that she has a memory problem and it's just about getting a wee bit more support. And one of the actual incidents that happened was the fall then she seemed to be very accepting of everything because they wanted to take her independence away.'

Barnes (2012) commented that independence is supported through autonomy and control and that dependence is managed through care and protection. The language of being independent is loaded with citizenship rights that can be denied to those deemed dependent (Brannelly, 2016). This could then be an example of Kate exploring the wider implications for her client of being labelled as *dependent* by others. This example also demonstrates the role of power in care planning where people are dependent on others to facilitate, or allow, their continued independence. Kate states that the care plan was accepted by the person concerned as she knew that the alternative was that 'they would take her independence away'. It is not explained why or how this would happen.

Expectations of Others
Re-Framing Resignation and Acceptance as Adjustment

Sometimes, support and care are provided to a person with dementia when they 'come to terms' with their present circumstances. These care plans are often practical and problem-solving in nature (as opposed to empowerment or resilience-based options) and form the basis for goal setting and reviews which follow. There can be examples of the needs of others being prioritised in this process. Implicit in all of this is the expectation that the person with dementia accepts that their life has changed, whether that is related to age, dementia or disability, and importantly that not to change or accept limitations would be problematic for those around the person.

Here, Gwen talks about her work with Alan, whom we met earlier:

'He does take in that he's having problems with certain things and he'll say things like, "Oh, my memory" and he does recognise that his wife has to do things and she'll say, "Remember that you have problems making something to eat" or do simple things like pick out his clothes. So, it's a case of trying to discuss that with him to say that, "You are struggling there." You know, helping him take that on board. You know, "This is what your wife's doing for you and she needs a break in the morning"… His involvement was about him coming to terms with what his wife actually does for him.'

Gwen states that Alan's role in the support-planning process is to *come to terms* with the care tasks that his wife undertakes. Gwen uses several phrases to emphasise this, such as 'he does take in' and 'he does recognise'. The account did not, however, reveal how the process of coming to terms would occur or what it would look like. This would appear to be an example of denying Alan's citizenship within the home. In the example below, from Doug, we can see that where the person with dementia doesn't accept the picture of self that is presented by other people, this can be positioned as the person being unrealistic. Österholm and Samuelsson (2014) identified that the social workers in their study positioned people with dementia as less competent than the other people present within the assessment interaction. There is then a risk of invalidating the person with dementia's opinion, where the person does not agree with the assessment findings, or the proposed support. This can be explained as a continued failure to recognise citizenship status and, as a result of this loss of recognition, the person concerned can be disempowered, even where, like Doug, the practitioner had tried to practice in an inclusive manner.

'A person with dementia who had a power of attorney, but the person doesn't realise how much the attorney is having to do or how much assistance she needs. They were going on holiday and she had to go to respite for a week as because of safety it was definitely worthwhile. So I did speak with her and write details in her diary and she was fine about it but on the day she didn't remember and she didn't want to go when the day came. She came round and I drove her there in my car and I could tell she wasn't herself and I didn't feel comfortable. But she couldn't be on her own, it was only for a week and I knew she would be looked after. I knew she didn't want to be there. So people with dementia can't always understand but for needs to be fully met…but I wasn't happy.'

Ian works with older people in a social care setting. He is working with Charles. He refers to Charles' roles as both husband and carer. However, the intervention appears to focus on Charles relinquishing aspects of these roles. There is no discussion about how important identities such as husband or carer might be supported through a resilience framework. This approach has the potential to result in further loss of identity for Charles and could result in loss of sense of self. Resilience could play a role in aligning outcomes that preserve identity, including those identities that contribute to the domestic sphere of citizenship as a core component. We need to remember that support can result in loss of roles, and loss of mastery and control, and that this can reduce resilience.

'He would limit what he did to ensure his wife's needs were met. He did articulate this to me but was very clear that was his role as a husband and was clear that he didn't want to change it too much. He didn't want to upset his wife and he didn't want her to say that he wasn't there for her... He was never resistant but was always quite clear that he had a role and he wasn't going to, kind of, be forced to take a back seat and that was very good to see that he could advocate for himself, advocate for his wife and had a clear idea about what he wanted... I think, the one thing that did come of this one, this assessment, although we recognised his commitment, his loyalty we actually had to work with him to move him away from some of those qualities because they were detrimental to him in that he would have went with his wife to a day service that wasn't suitable. He would have not, gained no benefit for himself. No rest from his caring role because he was quite definite about his need to be there and be the carer for his wife. For me it's about prioritising those needs and then being quite open with the client and saying, "This is what I'm thinking. This is what I propose. This is what I think I can do and this is how I see it working for you." We all practise in a way that's unique to us. That's the way I practise as it's something that I would want.'

What Can We Do?

The tensions between established knowledge of 'how people with dementia are', alongside attempts to work in a person-centred way with individuals, is an obstacle to working more creatively. Although many human service professionals want to work positively with the person with dementia, there do appear to be expectations that in order to move forward, the person has to accept limits or limitations in their new life as a person with dementia. This happens because of the fear that people with dementia are unable to judge risks, or are more at risk, due to the fact that the person has dementia. It happens because there are competing needs, carers are under immense pressure, and services have little in the way of support outside of respite, day care, home care, etc. It is, therefore, easier to work within the sphere of our existing practice knowledge, and predict likely outcomes based on the homogeneous group 'people with dementia'. It is also interesting that the independence of the person has such a central role in our practice. It is presented as an indicator of how well the person is 'coping' with their dementia; as a measure of how much support is required; and as motivation for intervention with independence being a desired outcome. Independence is, however, also discussed as a status to be granted or removed by others. This highlights the ways in which language and power go hand in hand.

Competing roles and priorities can affect how practitioners undertake work with people ageing with dementia. An emphasis on organisational objectives, process and resource provision can minimise opportunities to identify and promote resilience. Although this chapter has focused on tensions in practice, there are also many examples of value-based, reflective and thoughtful practice. However, without being mindful of the pitfalls, and having a consistent approach that identifies the potential for resilience, our practice can be tokenistic and may fall below expected standards. The next chapter will include some further examples of real-world applications.

CHAPTER 8

Realising Resilience

Practice Scenarios

This chapter presents an assortment of practice scenarios where a resilience focus has been adopted.

Jakub

Jakub lives on his own in a busy city centre. He retired from his work as a delivery driver five years ago, at the age of 70. He has never married and has no children. His brother lives in Poland with the rest of his extended family. Jakub has vascular dementia. Most of his friendships were work related. He doesn't go out much now, only to the shops for his paper in the morning. He has a community nurse, Mary, who visits. Mary is concerned that Jakub is lonely and at risk of isolation. If Mary employs a traditional problem-solving perspective she would focus on resources to combat loneliness, such as a referral to a day centre or a befriender. A resilience perspective starts with Jakub. Is he lonely? And if so, what are the reasons for this, what can be changed to enable him to feel less isolated, and what resources are needed to do this?

Resilience and Protective Factors

Jakub has lived on his own for a long time. He still has a morning routine of going to the shops and the shop owners, Phil and Linda, and staff know him. They would notice if didn't come for his paper. Jakub knows the family well as he has lived in his flat for over 30 years. He enjoys a morning catch-up on the local news when he is there. Jakub has grown used to retirement. He missed his work at first but has high blood pressure so was also relieved to retire. He found the hours long and the job could be stressful. He enjoys his current pace of life, although he does miss the conversation in his depot when he arrived back at the end of the shift. He is used to being on his own during the day as he travelled alone. Mary sees that Jakub has a sense of being connected to people and place. He has rewarding relationships with the local shop owner and family. He still feels like himself although an older, retired version of that self and he feels that he is doing okay. Jakub is resigned to his health problems and believes they are work related. He is generally happy with his lot in life. At home, he forgets to eat sometimes. Being on his own he only eats when he is hungry and recently he hasn't felt hungry very often. He isn't too worried about it although he has lost a little weight.

Mary makes the following Resilience Reserve notes:

Motivation: Jakub would like to have company but doesn't feel lonely.

Knowledge, skills and interests: Jakub knows the area well. He has a great memory for roads and journeys related to his work and loves to talk about different places.

Assets and resources: Own home, shop owner/friend, neighbours, local community.

Experiences: Jakub is used to his own company and is happy with his own company. He has a daily routine that suits him. The morning is much the same as it was before he retired, when he would make a cup of tea and sort out his travels for the day. He has always had a small circle of friends.

Roles: Driver, work colleague, neighbour, friend, brother, uncle.

Personal qualities: Sociable but on his own terms, helps out his neighbours when they need something.

Mary can see that Jakub is far more connected than she had realised at first. She creates a map with Jakub at the centre and lists all of the relationships that Jakub has and the daily contacts that he has. He is in touch with his brother who calls once a week. Mary is, however, concerned that Jakub's confidence in his home routine is leaving him vulnerable to missing meals unless she supports him to put some structure around this. She puts a notepad in the kitchen beside the kettle with a reminder for Jakub to check the fridge for his lunch that day. With Jakub's agreement they also both speak to Phil and Linda, who agree to prompt Jakub about his lunch when he sees them in the morning. They will also check that Jakub has shopping in. Mary and Jakub have a chat about him going out to a local café or community group for lunch. There is a local hobby group that meets to go walking. Although Jakub isn't sure about this, the group discuss the local area and other travels when they meet and so Mary thinks it is a good fit. Jakub agrees to meet with the walk leader to see if it will suit him.

Jane and William

Jane and William have been married for over 50 years. They met when William was in the army and Jane was working on a local farm. Jane raised their two daughters, Sara and Jill, before she took a job in the hospitality sector at a local hotel and is now retired. They both describe their family life as happy, enjoying the outdoors and meeting with friends. Jane is a member of a local art group and William is a keen golfer. Lately, however, William has not been able to play golf as regularly as he would like. He has arthritis and playing golf is now difficult. He misses the social side of going to the club as he would talk to his friends as they walked around the course about what was happening at home.

Jane has recently been confused about things in the home, forgetting where she put her purse or how the cooker works. William hadn't worried too much about this as he put it down to old age, but just yesterday, Jane couldn't remember his name. Willian also received a call to tell him that Jane had not turned up for her art group. She was later found at the local hotel having reported for work. He is now frightened to leave her on her own. William has noticed that Jane has been wearing the same clothes for several days which she never did before. He hasn't told his daughters about his concerns as he doesn't want to worry them. William shares his concerns about his wife when he visits the doctor's surgery for pain relief related to his arthritis. His GP arranges for Fathimaa, a link worker, to visit to see if she can help.

Resilience and Protective Factors

Fathimaa spends time getting to know both Jane and William. She can see that they are a close couple and that William is struggling to accept that Jane might need some more support. William doesn't want to admit that things are changing and finds this difficult to talk about. Looking at the resilience of both parties as well as the ways in which the wellbeing of one affects the other is key. The biggest worry is that Jane had been lost. So, they start by talking about this. Jane doesn't remember what happened but laughs about the story when William recalls it. They all agree that they don't know that Jane got lost, only that she went to the hotel mistakenly for her work. Jane has William, she has friends and she has interests. When she didn't arrive at the group she was missed and William was able to act. Jane blames her memory loss on having such a demanding job at the hotel where she had to remember lots of things and manage lots of people. She loved the responsibility but thinks that now she has retired her brain has slowed down. She isn't worried about this. Jane feels that she is doing okay. William is stressed about the situation. He finds Jane's lack of concern frustrating as he can't seem to make her understand how serious he feels the situation might have been.

Fathimaa begins to populate a Resilience Reserve with Jane. She feels this will also help William to see that Jane has lots of resources to draw on. Her notes include:

Motivation: Jane wants to meet friends and continue to go to her art group.

Knowledge, skills and interests: Jane has a talent for art and is very creative. She is organised and used to managing lots of things at the same time. She is a people person and liked by others.

Assets and resources: Friends, family, comfortable home and finances, nice neighbourhood, lots of local amenities. William is looking out for her and she can confide in him.

Experiences: Jane was a manager of a busy hotel and a mother. She is used to problem solving and juggling demands.

Roles: Mother, manager, friend, wife.

Personal qualities: Great sense of humour, loves looking after others and can be relied on by her family and friends. She describes herself as stubborn at times and likes to be independent.

Fathimaa also uses the Quick Rating Tool to summarise the situation (see Table 8.1).

Table 8.1 Fathimaa's Quick Rating of Risk and Protective Factors

Protective Factors	Score Protective Factors 1–5 **Strongly Agree 5** **Agree 4** **Mostly Agree 3** **Disagree 2** **Strongly Disagree 1**	Risk Factors
Sense of being connected to people and places *Comments:* *Jane scores really highly in this category and has lots of resources to draw on.*	Rewarding relationships with others *Score: 5* Sense of belonging *Score: 5* I still feel like me *Score: 5*	Isolation/ disconnectedness *Comments:*

Sense of mastery and control, self-efficacy and self-esteem	Feels able to influence events and people in his or her life	Loss of mastery and control, self-efficacy, self-esteem
Comments:	*Score: 4*	*Comments:*
Jane is confident that she can deal with issues that arise. An example is that she did 'report' to her old place of work when she didn't go to her art group and her husband was called.	Is confident in self if a problem arises *Score: 4* Feels good about self or achievements in life *Score: 5*	
Meaning making	I feel that I am doing okay	No meaning making/lack of opportunity for meaning making
Comments:	*Score: 4*	*Comments:*
Jane feels that she has slowed down since she retired and that her memory is worse because of this.	My life makes sense to me *Score: 4*	

Jane has lots of protective factors and is at low risk of the negative impact of dementia. Fathimaa completes the same exercise for William (Table 8.2).

Table 8.2 Fathimaa's Quick Rating of Risk and Protective Factors (Carer)

Protective Factors	Score Protective Factors 1–5 Strongly Agree 5 Agree 4 Mostly Agree 3 Disagree 2 Strongly Disagree 1	Risk Factors
Sense of being connected to people and places *Comments:* *William is finding his time with me as supportive and is talking freely about his worries.*	Rewarding relationships with others *Score: 2* Sense of belonging *Score: 4* I still feel like me *Score: 3*	Isolation/ disconnectedness *Comments:* *William doesn't see his friends at the golf. This is where he would talk. He doesn't want to go out and leave Jane alone and so is further isolating himself.* *William doesn't want to tell his daughters what is happening and has been distancing himself and Jane from regular family contact.*
Sense of mastery and control, self-efficacy and self-esteem *Comments:* *Although Willian didn't know what to do he spoke to his GP for advice.*	Feels able to influence events and people in his or her life *Score: 2* Is confident in self if a problem arises *Score: 3* Feels good about self or achievements in life *Score: 4*	Loss of mastery and control, self-efficacy, self-esteem *Comments:* *William feels that he has little control over the situation due to Jane's dementia. He was frightened when she didn't go to her art club as planned.*

Meaning making Comments: *William is confused about what is happening to Jane but puts his health problems and Jane's down to old age. He is working through issues with me when we meet and learning about dementia.*	I feel that I am doing okay *Score: 3* My life makes sense to me *Score: 3*	No meaning making/lack of opportunity for meaning making Comments:

William, however, appears to be struggling with the changes. To some extent, Jane has always managed things at home. He has begun to isolate himself from others. He is not going to his golf club and he hasn't spoken to his daughters. When they look at this together they identify three areas of action.

1. To see how Jane's need for independence and William's need for her to be safe can be met.

2. To enhance William's connections and support network.

3. To help him regain some sense of control over circumstances.

They arrange for one of Jane's friends to call for her and they go to the art group venue together. William also agrees to talk to his daughters about what has been happening. William's pain relief for his arthritis is reviewed and he starts to go to the golf clubhouse when Jane is at her group. As a family, they agree to re-visit the arrangements if Jane gets 'lost' again but William is reassured that Jane went to a place she knew well and reminds himself that his wife has always been a resourceful woman. This exercise has helped him to see that Jane still has a lot of experience to draw on even if he can't always understand her actions. Fathimaa also explores ways to help Jane maintain her interests, and address any new concerns as they arise with the local occupational therapy team.

Sunil and Lottie

Sunil is a social worker in a city hospital. He has been working with Lottie who is 90 years old. Lottie was admitted to hospital with a chest infection. She has Alzheimer's disease. Sunil is undertaking an assessment of need as Lottie is now ready to leave hospital. Concerns have been expressed by family members that Lottie is not managing at home. She has a pet dog, Max, that her son is currently looking after. Sunil has noted that Lottie appears very low. Her confidence has been knocked by her fall and she misses Max.

Sunil uses the Resilience Reserve to begin to map all of the different resources that Lottie has access to at home. He also uses intersectionality to consider the ways in which the current hospital environment might be preventing Lottie from accessing these resources. Intersectionality helps us understand the aspects of our life in which we have power and those where we experience disempowerment and discrimination. So, for example, Max plays a big part in Lottie's life at home. He is a source of affection and she finds looking after him very rewarding. Lottie loves her daily walking routine with Max and meets fellow dog walkers when she is out. In hospital she doesn't have routine, connections or the freedoms of home. Using the Risk and Protective Factors Quick Rating Tool, Sunil can see that Lottie's scores are lower in hospital than they would be at home. Sunil arranges Lottie's discharge, liaising with her family, Lottie's GP and the local social services department. Lottie has a home support worker who visits once a week. Sunil shares the Resilience Reserve outline and his analysis of the risk and protective factors that contribute to Lottie's wellbeing. As a result, Lottie's relationship with Max and her activities related to looking after Max are prioritised as important aspects of her support planning. There is also a re-ablement team in Lottie's area. Sunil speaks to them about any support that could be available to Lottie to reduce the likelihood of another fall.

Colin

Colin is 86 years old. He and his wife, Rena, were living apart due to her admission to a local care home. Both Colin and his wife have Alzheimer's disease. Colin reluctantly agreed to his wife moving to care as his family believed this to be the best option. He spends all of his free time with Rena at the care home as it is within walking distance of the marital home. Colin has had his diagnosis for over two years. He was his wife's carer for ten years. The care home staff are concerned about Colin. He is dressed smartly and always likes to wear a shirt and tie, but now his clothes are noticeably dirty with food stains. Colin is unshaven and his hair is uncombed which is at odds with his appearance generally. Colin would usually shave every day. The manager of the care home, Tanya, tries to speak to Colin to see how he is but he just replies that everything is fine. She decides to speak to Colin's son when he next visits Rena and he agrees that things appear to have deteriorated at home for Colin; however, he won't accept any help and won't listen when his son tries to speak to him. Tanya agrees to support the family in trying to talk to Colin. Tanya asks Colin about how he is feeling about the situation.

> 'I can't remember what's been happening really. My wife has always been very active until you know. Was she in hospital? Oh yes, but not very long just in and out. I think she could remember things far back and I think that happens with people with this. She could forget wee ordinary things about the house, you know? What she has been talking about or people's name or things like that. Oh, she still knows the family. She's not too bad.'

Colin doesn't refer to his own experience of dementia and instead talks about his wife and her own health. His story reveals contradictions. He and his wife had experienced her decline into ill-health, hospital care and she had moved to a care home setting. However, Colin's view is that things aren't that bad. He could be minimising the impact of dementia on himself, his wife and his life. He avoids any discussion that challenges his world view and despite the major changes in his living arrangements Colin maintains that everything in his life is fine. This appears to be a self-protecting mechanism. Colin denies that dementia has had an impact on him or his life. So, despite significant changes Colin has adopted a fixed approach to the situation. There is little evidence of adaptation which is the key feature of resilience, or any adjustments in the face of adversity. Tanya concludes that Colin is vulnerable to the impact of dementia as the condition progresses as he appears fixed on a 'nothing is wrong' approach. This is despite the strain of responding to his wife's care needs, and the physical changes that Tanya can see in Colin. She makes a referral to the local social work department at the request of the family as they will need support to plan for the future and

Colin needs to spend time with someone who will get to know him and address his own needs moving forward.

Maura

Maura lives in sheltered housing. She has been living with dementia for three years. She has been having some difficulty finding her way around the building and has been trying to enter her neighbour's apartment. Her neighbor, Joan, has health issues of her own and she understandably gets upset when she hears someone trying to come into her home. Paul, who is the complex manager, doesn't know what to do for the best. He has tried talking to Maura about it but she is annoyed when he does. Maura doesn't have any family and Paul is worried that things will become worse. He knows that people with dementia can 'wander'. Joan's family have already complained to him.

Paul can use resilience to approach the problem from Maura's perspective. In doing this he is moving from a 'people with dementia' to 'this person living with dementia' perspective. He invites Maura to walk around the building with him on a couple of occasions over the week as he goes about his work. This gives them the opportunity to chat as they walk. Paul can find out more about Maura and they can talk about a wide range of interests without it feeling like a 'meeting' where Paul is raising concerns. Maura had been a volunteer before she moved into the complex. She enjoyed helping people and found it very rewarding. Paul didn't know this and was surprised at how animated Maura was when she discussed her work. As they walk he notices how Maura relies on cues within the built environment when she can't recall how to get back to her apartment. He also sees that the doors to the apartments are similar, distinguishable only by numbers. Maura tells him her address at her previous home where she stayed for most of her life. She doesn't recall her apartment number here. There is a pot plant at the end of the corridor and Maura uses this as a prompt that she is on the right floor. However, she can't remember which apartment is hers and, as a result, can sometimes try Joan's door with her key.

Resilience and Protective Factors

Paul now has a better insight into what motivates Maura. Using the Resilience Reserve, he creates a visual record of Maura's assets and resources. She wants to help others and she gets a great deal from doing this. He also identifies the ways in which both the built and social environment might be disabling Maura. Paul takes advice on dementia enabling design and works with Maura to make her own apartment door more identifiable to her. He also asks Maura if she would be happy to talk at a dementia awareness event. Maura was delighted to be asked and Paul arranges a small discussion evening for staff, tenants and families who want to come. He also invites the local Alzheimer's organisation. Maura meets with them in advance and they plan a slot for her to talk about her volunteering and her experience of dementia.

In this example, Paul has moved out of his comfort zone and tried a different approach to see an issue from the perspective of the person with dementia. Maura is supported through changes to the building design and she feels valued by the invitation to share her experiences, not just of living with dementia, but her life experiences. This offers her opportunities to make new connections, retain a sense of mastery and control, and make sense of who she is now.

Summary

The varied examples provided in this chapter on practice scenarios provide a glimpse into the ways in which resilience can inform our practice. Resilience approaches can be used by a wide range of practitioners, in a variety of settings, to help us better understand the person and the problem from their perspective. In the final chapter we will, therefore, ask 'Where to from here?'

CHAPTER 9

The Road to Resilience

Where to from Here?

I want to start this final chapter by reflecting on what's important. Every person living with dementia is important. Their lives and experiences are too. His or her relationships and sense of self are important. So too is the everyday work of the people that provide support. Our work, which is essentially intervening in people's story of self, is the difference between supporting a sense of continuity or indirectly facilitating disconnectedness from self and others. Identity and self-recognition are achieved through the quiet, often ordinary, rhythm of life. Our everyday activities are the foundations of identity. They are important. Challenges are part of life. Responding and adapting to the challenges of life is part of this process. Resilience can, therefore, be thought of as the background mechanism which keeps our story on track as we live this life. It is hard then to imagine how we can work with people living with dementia and carers without thinking about resilience. And once you begin to, you can see it all around, including its influence in your own life and the lives of those closest to you.

What Have We Learned?

What have we learned in our exploration of resilience in the context of dementia? People ageing with dementia have the potential for resilience. This is supported by the potential for cognitive (Clare *et al.*, 2011), motivational (Forstmeier and Maercker, 2008) and intersectional (Hulko, 2009) reserves. In order to understand this, we have to first reflect on the nature of life with dementia, of holding on to self despite changing circumstances. For some people this is easier as he or she will have protective factors that lessen the impact. Other people, who don't have this same access to buffers, will struggle in the face of changes and will be at risk of losing self, or aspects of self, as 'dementia' becomes the thing that most defines them. If we can recognise the factors that make this difference we can then judge the potential risk of loss of self and the buffers that need to be built up or built on. We can refer to each person's Resilience Reserve to find resources, or we can provide resources on a long or short-term basis. Re-ablement, rehabilitation and technology can all play a part in this.

Resilience is not called 'ordinary magic' (Masten, 2001) for nothing. People use resilience all of the time. However, unlike other people, those with dementia can find their resilient responses misinterpreted or re-labelled by others (Hughes *et al.*, 2006). If the resilience of the person with dementia is to be realised it must first be recognised by those engaged in practice and interaction with the individual concerned. This happens within relationships but is dependent on three factors. First, that carers and practitioners recognise reflections of identity within the stories told by people with dementia. The ways in which stories unfold could be an expression of resilience strategies in the preservation of identity. Second, that we understand the significance of these reflections within a resilience context. Placing these stories within a continuum of protective and vulnerability factors might enable practitioners to see the person as a citizen, family member, as a member of their community, alongside other important assessment data to reveal resilience and promote critical analysis. This change in perspective, from a person in need of service, to a citizen with assets and resources, is necessary to hear stories which are important pieces of the resilience jigsaw. Finally, that the concept of the resilience of the person with dementia is incorporated into a wider social understanding of every person unique to their individual situation. Our own stories about the people with dementia that we work with are also important. An awareness of the ways in which practice is described, and how these descriptions are used as a means of persuasion, could reveal potential opportunities and challenges to realising citizenship and resilience, in everyday practice. The opportunity to visualise resilience and Resilience Reserve could be a powerful tool for people with dementia to use to communicate their own needs in interaction with others. Problem solving, empowerment and asset-based work could then become the norm.

Resilience as a Window into Life with Dementia

Initially, when I started I was focused on defining resilience in the lives of people with dementia and answering the question: can people with dementia be resilient? However, I began to realise that what was important was what resilience taught me about dementia and life with dementia. I have been humbled by the intimate nature of stories that people willingly share about self, society and observations on life. The stories told by people with dementia can be dismissed as non-factual or superficial, assumed to have no substance or purpose (Sabat, 2006; Young, 2010). However, I found that the stories told by people ageing with dementia can in fact be rich reflections on life. In particular, stories can reveal insights into what might constitute a better than expected life for that particular individual, and without that story, this can remain hidden from view. What a waste. Stories are, therefore, powerful and at the same time sensitive and must be treated with respect. This applies to the act of generating stories together, but also to the handling of stories entrusted to us, as they are transformed into assessment content or data for analysis. Stories offer points of reflection and re-positioning for people. The active nature of this approach allows the person to possibly regain power within interactions, and so resilience has an opportunity to flourish.

Reflecting on this further, the act of storytelling, in and of itself, can provide an opportunity for resilience to be realised. Invitations to tell stories, and the knowledge that we are curious and willing to listen, can be a catalyst for resilience to be realised. Opportunities for reflections on the experience of practice through storytelling could possibly offer something new that would benefit both the practitioner in their ongoing professional development, and ultimately the person that we are engaged with. Storyboards offer a new dynamic in understanding layers of potentially hidden narrative. This can be a very accessible practice tool with which to engage with the stories of people with dementia and/or as part of an assessment process. My experience of using storyboards has led me to believe that this is an under-used resource that could be of interest to human service professionals both in their practice and in the communication of their practice with others.

The Resilience of the Dementia Network

Of course, it is not only the resilience of the person with dementia that is important. The support and wellbeing of carers is also an essential part of the equation. This book has focused on the resilience of the person with dementia particularly because there has been so much work (deservedly so) on promoting the resilience of carers. You can use the Resilience Reserve model in work with carers, as well as work with the person with dementia, and indeed, in doing so, it provides an opportunity to compare factors within caring and interdependent dyads. It also provides an opportunity to look at the pooled resources within care partnerships. Where resources can be shared, this model provides an opportunity to use resilience to further strengthen the shared experience of finding ways to cope. Where there are differences, this model can help carers gain an insight into why the person with dementia is responding in the way they are.

Similarly, practitioners and support staff can also use this model to explore their own resilience as part of reflecting on role and practice. What is adversity in the context of human service practitioners? Stressful events upset our emotional equilibrium and can lead to feelings of distress. Our work involves emotional labour so we need to recognise feelings of distress and that we need time to reflect and restore our emotional balance. Clear boundaries are also required to prevent over-empathising and over-involvement. Where communication issues feature it can sometimes feel like relationships, which are the bedrock of our practice, are difficult to achieve. Practitioners can also be subject to verbal and physical assaults in the course of their work. A study into the effects of verbal abuse on nurses, for example, found that verbalisations which are targeted, demeaning or humiliating were associated with anger responses, more so than being on the receiving end of physical assault (Jalil *et al.*, 2017). Organisational and socio-political factors also cause us distress or fail to recognise the need to make space to talk about the emotional labour of the job and of life. We explored this in Chapter 7. We can feel less able to deal with work if there are other things happening in our lives which are causing us distress. This can mean that we are then less available to the people that we work with. If this continues over time it can cause distress and burn-out.

Again, this model can be used from an organisational perspective to support the importance of resilience in the work of human service professionals. We can support ourselves and our staff by developing a culture of resilience. This involves creating space and time to reflect on your own resilience and sense of wellbeing. Reflection facilitates an awareness of feelings and beliefs. During supervision, expressing and questioning doubts, values and assumptions can help us to reach decisions in complex situations. This helps us develop co-operative problem-solving and decision-making abilities. To know that you are not alone but are part of a team can be a powerful thing.

We can do this by developing resilience toolkits. To start, complete your own Resilience Reserve to see the resources you have access to personally and within your organisation. Colleagues can also choose to do this collectively and within teams. Take a temperature reading of your wellbeing. How do you feel in the moment? Why might this be? The Quick Rating Tool can also help focus your thoughts here. We can think then about what would help you to improve your own wellbeing, how you support others, how you are supported in turn, and what resources you have access to that can act as buffers in the face of current difficulties. This toolkit can then be used in supervision, mentorship, peer support and reflective spaces. Reflective thinking skills and ways of being are, therefore, important. There is also a place for practical tools for stress management, mindfulness and relaxation. Remembering that *we* are a resource for our colleagues in difficult times is also part of a supportive work culture.

Concluding Remarks

The potential of the person to continue to grow and develop is at the heart of assessing resilience. However, in order to understand experience in the face of adversity it is important to listen carefully to what the person we are working with tells us about everyday life with dementia. This means leaving assumptions and pre-conceptions at the door. Only by doing this can we realise resilience through our practice. A resilience discourse can facilitate a re-conceptualisation of work with people ageing with dementia and, as a result, offer new opportunities to realise resilient identities through practice, education and research. It can do this in the following ways:

- Applying a resilience discourse to the subject of identity and dementia can reveal new insights and offer alternative perspectives on both dementia and the nature of resilience itself.

- The stories told by people ageing with dementia can be demonstrations of resilience in action performed by social citizens.

- New opportunities to realise resilient identities will occur through defining resilience in the context of ageing with dementia; visualising the possibility of a Resilience Reserve; and developing, and using, a resilience framework in practice, education and research settings.

In conclusion, we all have the potential for resilience no matter our age or circumstances. Resilience is not static and is influenced by the complex interaction of vulnerability and protective factors. When a person has dementia, resilience is an important factor in the preservation of identity and holding on to sense of self. Yet, practitioners do not readily use frameworks that facilitate resilience in work with people ageing with dementia. With such a framework, practice and research with people ageing with dementia can then take place, within a new model of citizenship that recognises the contributions that people with dementia make to their own lives, and to those of other people. Recognising the potential for resilience in people living with dementia does not mean ignoring the needs of carers or minimising risks or concerns. Working with care networks is an important part of supporting resilience infrastructure. Resilience has real-world applications and as such these complexities need to be reflected.

It is important to remember that not everyone living with dementia will be 'resilient' and not everyone is resilient in every situation. Neither is a focus on resilience an excuse to ignore risks or concerns or our statutory responsibilities to people in need. Resilience is a fluid, complicated concept. However, applying the resilience model outlined in this book will help practitioners to navigate these complexities whilst keeping the person at the heart of the process. This places resilience in a continuum of real-world practice where we can intervene by helping the person to employ assets and resources, and providing resources where they are needed. People living with dementia are individuals with different lives, different life experiences, skills, knowledge and expertise. Dementia does not erode our personhood or our life experiences and to ignore this is to under-utilise a valuable repository of personal assets and resources which could be supported and employed in helping people adjust to life with dementia. Equally, resilience helps us to understand the ways in which our own attitudes, practices and approach could undermine the identity of the person with dementia. I, therefore, conclude that the concept of resilience can contribute much to our understanding of dementia. However, how people experience dementia and respond to the challenges of living with dementia can also reveal much about the nature of resilience. Our lives are stories in motion, and so, in turning our attention to resilience, let us create better stories of living with dementia together.

Glossary

Adversity: a difficult or unpleasant situation. This can be a single event or over a period of time.

Asset: a useful or valuable item or thing that a person possesses.

Cognitive reserve: theory that the brain finds different ways to respond to loss of function by employing reserves from another area.

Connectedness: a feeling of belonging to a person, group, place or thing.

Co-production: citizens, statutory services and organisations making the best use of each other's knowledge, skills, experiences, assets and resources to achieve an objective. Addressing power imbalance is central to co-production and sets it apart from participation.

Identity: the distinguishing personality of an individual: who he or she is and is known to be.

Ill-being: an absence of wellbeing; lack of happiness; state of unease.

Interdependence: the dependence of two or more people on each other or things.

Intersectionality: the interconnected nature of social categories such as race, class and gender creating overlapping and interdependent systems of discrimination or disadvantage, and promoting areas of privilege.

Mastery and control: knowledge, skill and autonomy; (sense of) the feeling that you have knowledge, skills and autonomy.

Meaning making: the process of how persons construe, understand or make sense of life events, relationships and the self.

Motivation: a reason or purpose for acting, or behaving, in a particular way.

Protective factors: people, things or circumstances which decrease the likelihood of a negative outcome (harm) and make a positive outcome more likely.

Resilience: the process of adaptation in the face of adversity. In the context of dementia, resilience can be thought of as the process of *adaptation to hold on to a sense of self in the face of threats to identity.*

Resilience domains: topic areas that together constitute the Resilience Reserve.

Resilience matrix: an overview of resilience in the context of dementia. It illustrates the intersection of identity and risk in the experience of dementia and the role of protective and risk factors.

Resilience Reserve: a personal repository of resources consisting of six resilience domains. It is this repository that we refer to when responding to the challenges that we face.

Resources: a stock or supply of materials, items, connections and other assets that can be drawn on by a person in order to function effectively.

Risk: a situation involving exposure to danger or harm.

Risk factors: people or circumstances that contribute to exposure to danger or harm.

Salutogenesis: theory which highlights the factors that promote health rather than those that cause disease. (It is closely linked to asset-based approaches.)

Sense of self: the feeling that one's identity is in keeping with the self-image held. A sense of continuity that the self is constant over time.

Storyboard: a sequence of drawings or headings which lay out the trajectory of a story or discussion. This illuminates the smaller stories that make up the larger whole.

Threat: a person or thing likely to cause damage or danger.

Vulnerable: exposed to the possibility of being harmed.

Vulnerability factors: people, things and circumstances which increase the likelihood of a negative outcome (harm) and make a positive outcome less likely.

Wellbeing: the state of being comfortable, healthy and happy.

Bibliography

Abbema, R.V., Bielderman, A., De Greef, M., Hobbelen, H., Krijnen, W. and Van der Schans, C. (2015) Building from a conceptual model of the resilience process during ageing. Towards the Groningen Aging Resilience Inventory. *Journal of Advanced Nursing,* 71 (9): 2208–2219.

Allen, R.S., Haley, P.P., Harris, G.M., Fowler, S.N. and Roopwinder, P. (2011) Resilience: Definitions, Ambiguities and Applications. In: B. Resnick, L.P. Gwyther and K.A. Roberto (eds) *Resilience in Aging: Concepts, Research and Outcomes.* New York: Springer.

Althusser, L. (1971) *Lenin and Philosophy and Other Essays.* London: New Left Books.

Alzheimer Disease International (2018) *The State of the Art of Dementia Research. New Frontiers.* Available at www.alz.co.uk/research/WorldAlzheimerReport2018.pdf (accessed February 2019).

Antonovsky, A. (1979) *Health, Stress, and Coping: New Perspectives on Physical and Mental Well-being.* San Francisco, CA: Jossey-Bass.

Antonovsky, A. (1987) *Unravelling the Mystery of Health: How People Manage Stress and Stay Well.* San Francisco, CA: Jossey-Bass.

Antonovsky, A. (1991) The structural sources of salutogenic strengths. In: C.L. Cooper and R. Payne (eds) *Personality and Stress: Individual Differences in the Stress Process.* New York: John Wiley.

Bailey, C., Clarke, C.L., Gibb, C., Haining, S., Wilkinson, H. and Tiplady, S. (2013) Risky and resilient life with dementia: Review of and reflections on the literature. *Health, Risk and Society,* 10: 1–10.

Baldwin, C. (2008) Narrative(,) citizenship and dementia: The personal and the political. *Journal of Aging Studies,* 22 (3): 222–228.

Barnes, R., Auburn, T. and Lea, S. (2004) Citizenship in Practice. *British Journal of Social Psychology,* 43: 187–206.

Barnes, M. (2012) *Care in Everyday Life.* Bristol: University Press.

Barry, M. (2007) *Effective Approaches to Risk Assessment in Social Work: An International Literature Review. Social Research Findings No 31.* Edinburgh: Scottish Executive Education Department.

Bartlett, R. and O'Connor, D. (2007) From Personhood to Citizenship: Broadening the lens for dementia practice and research. *Journal of Aging Studies*, 21: 107–118.

Bartlett, R. (2016) Scanning the conceptual horizons of citizenship. *Dementia*, 15 (3): 453–461.

Batsch, N. and Mittelman, S. (2012) *Alzheimer Disease International. World Alzheimer Report. Overcoming the Stigma of Dementia*. London: ADI.

Bavidge, M. (2006) Ageing and Human Nature. In: J.C. Hughes, S.J. Louw and S.R. Sabat (eds) *Dementia: Mind, Meaning and the Person*. Oxford: Oxford University Press.

Bennett, K.M. (2010) How to achieve resilience as an older widower: Turning points or gradual change? *Ageing and Society*, 30 (3): 369–382.

Berger, P.L and Luckman, T. (1966) *The Social Construction of Reality*. New York: Doubleday.

Brannelly, T. (2016) Citizenship and people living with dementia: A case for the ethics of care. *Dementia*, 15 (3): 304–314.

Bowes, A. and Daniel, B. (2010) Interrogating harm and abuse: A lifespan approach. *Social Policy and Society*, 9 (2): 221–229.

Bowlby, J. (1980) *Attachment and Loss: Loss, Sadness and Depression: Volume 3*. New York: Basic Books.

Bowlby, J. (1982) *Attachment and Loss: Volume 1. Attachment*. New York: Basic Books.

Bowlby, J. (1988) *A Secure Base: Parent–Child Attachment and Healthy Human Development*. New York: Basic Books.

Bowling, A. and Dieppe, P. (2005) What is successful ageing and who should define it? *British Medical Journal*, 331: 1548–1551.

Bubeck, D. (1995) *Care, Gender and Justice*. Oxford: Clarendon Press.

Butler, R.N. (1963) The Life Review: An interpretation of reminiscence in the aged. *Psychiatry, Journal for the Study of Inter-personal Processes*, 26. Reprinted in: B.L. Neugarten (ed.) (1968) *Middle Age and Aging*. Chicago: University of Chicago Press.

Butler, R. (1969) Age-ism: Another form of bigotry. *The Gerontologist*, 9 (4): 243–246.

Caddell, L. and Clare, L. (2010) The impact of dementia on self and identity: A systematic review. *Clinical Psychology Review*, 30: 113–126.

Caddell, L. and Clare, L. (2011) Studying the self in people with dementia: How might we proceed? *Dementia*, 12 (2): 192–209.

Cations, M., May, N., Crotty, M., Low, L-F., Clemson, L., Whitehead, C., McLoughlin, J., Swaffer, K. and Laver, K.E. (2019) Health professional perspectives on rehabilitation for people with dementia. *The Gerontologist*, gnz007, https://doi.org/10.1093/geront/gnz007.

Charon, J.M. (1992) *Symbolic Interactionism: An Introduction, An Interpretation, An Integration. Fourth Edition*. New Jersey: Prentice-Hall Inc.

Chandler, D. and Reid, J. (2016) *The Neoliberal Subject: Resilience, Adaptation and Vulnerability*. London: Rowman and Littlefield International.

Clare, L. (2003) Managing threats to self: Awareness in the early stage of Alzheimer's disease. *Social Science & Medicine*, 57: 1017–1029.

Clare, L. and Shakespeare, P. (2004) Negotiating the impact of forgetting: Dimensions of resistance in task-orientated conversations between people with early stage dementia and their partners. *Dementia*, 3: 211–232.

Clare, L., Kinden, D.E.J., Woods, R.T., Whitaker, R. *et al.* (2010) Goal-orientated cognitive rehabilitation for people with early-stage Alzheimer disease: A single-bind randomized controlled trial of clinical efficacy. *The American Journal of Geriatric Psychiatry*, 18 (10): 928–939.

Clare, L., Kinsella, G.J., Logsdon, R., Whitlatch, C. and Zarit, S.H. (2011) Building Resilience in Mild Cognitive Impairment and Early-Stage Dementia: Innovative Approaches to Intervention and Outcome Evaluation. In: B. Resnick, L.O. Gwyther and K. Roberto (eds) *Resilience in Aging: Concepts, Research and Outcomes*. New York: Springer.

Clare, L., Wu, Y.T., Teale, J.C., MacLeod, C., Matthews, F., Brayne, C., Woods, B. and CFAS-Wales study team (2017) Potentially modifiable lifestyle factors, cognitive reserve, and cognitive function in later life: A cross-sectional study. *PLOS Med* 14, 3 (online article) doi:10.1371/journal.pmed.1002259 (accessed February 2019).

Clark, P.G., Burbank, P.M., Greene, G. Owens, N. and Riebe, D. (2011) What Do We Know About Resilience in Older Adults? An Exploration of Some Facts, Factors and Facets. In: B. Resnick, L.O. Gwyther and K. Roberto (eds) *Resilience in Aging: Concepts, Research and Outcomes*. New York: Springer.

Clarke, C.L. and Bailey, C. (2016) Narrative citizenship, resilience and inclusion with dementia: On the inside or on the outside of physical and social places. *Dementia*, 15 (3): 434–452.

Clarke, C.L., Keady, J., Wilkinson, H., Gibb, C.E., Luce, A., Cook, A. and Williams, L. (2010) Dementia and risk: Contested territories of everyday life. *Journal of Nursing and Healthcare of Chronic Illness*, 2 (2): 102–112.

Coulshed, V. and Orme, J. (1998) *Social Work Practice: An Introduction. Third Edition*. Hampshire: Palgrave.

Cox, S., Anderson, I., Dick, S. and Elgar, J. (1998) *The Person, the Community and Dementia: Developing a Value Framework*. Stirling: Dementia Development Centre, University of Stirling.

Crenshaw-Williams, K. (1989) Demarginalising the intersection of race and sex: A black feminist critique of antidiscrimination doctrine, feminist theory and antiracist politics. *University of Chicago Legal Forum*, 1: 139–167.

Cuddy, A.J., Norton, M.I. and Fiske, S.T. (2005) 'This old stereotype': The pervasiveness and persistence of the elderly stereotype. *Journal of Social Issues*, 61 (2): 267–285.

Daniel, B. and Wassell, S. (2002a) *The Early Years: Assessing and Promoting Resilience in Vulnerable Children 1*. London: Jessica Kingsley Publishers.

Daniel, B and Wassell, S. (2002b) *The School Years: Assessing and Promoting Resilience in Vulnerable Children 2*. London: Jessica Kingsley Publishers.

Daniel, B and Wassell, S. (2002c) *Adolescence: Assessing and Promoting Resilience in Vulnerable Children 3*. London: Jessica Kingsley Publishers.

De Beauvoir, S. (1977) *Old Age*. Middlesex: Penguin Books.

Department of Health (2012) *Prime Minister's Challenge on Dementia. Delivering Major Improvements in Dementia Care and Research by 2015*. London. Department of Health.

Dias, R., Santos, R.L., Sousa, M.F., Torres, B., Belfort, T. and Dourado, M.C. (2015) Resilience of caregivers of people with dementia: A systematic review of biological and psychosocial determinants. *Trends in Psychiatry and Psychotherapy*, 37 (1): 12–19.

Erikson, E.H. (1965) *Childhood and Society*. New York: Norton.

Erikson. E.H. (1968) *Identity, Youth and Crisis*. New York. Norton.

Erikson, E.H. (1980) *Identity and the Lifecycle*. New York: Norton.

European Court of Human Rights (2010) *European Convention on Human Rights*. Council of Europe. Available at www.echr.coe.int/Documents/Convention_ENG.pdf (accessed February 2019).

Forstmeier, S. and Maercker, A. (2008) Motivational Reserve: Lifetime motivational abilities contribute to cognitive and emotional health in old age. *Psychology and Aging*, 23 (4): 886–899.

Fricker, M. (2007) *Epistemic Injustice: Power and the Ethics of Knowing*. Oxford: Oxford University Press.

Friedland, R., Fritsch, T., Smyth, K.A., Koss, E., Lerner. A. J., Hsuin-Chen, C., Petot, G.J. and Debanne, S.M. (2001) Patients with Alzheimer's disease have reduced activities in midlife compared with healthy control-group members. *Proceedings of the National Academy of Sciences of the United States of America*, 98 (6): 3440–3445.

Garmezy, N. (1974) The study of competence in children at risk for severe psychopathology. In: E.J. Anthony and C. Koupernik (eds) *The Child in his Family: Children at Psychiatric Risk III*. New York: Wylie.

Giebel, C.M. and Sutcliffe, C. (2017) Initiating activities of daily living contributes to well-being in people with dementia and their carers. *International Journal of Geriatric Psychiatry*, 33, 1. http://doi.org/10.1002/gps.4728 (accessed February 2019).

Goffman, E. (1959) *The Presentation of Self in Everyday Life*. London: Routledge.

Goffman, E. (1963) *Stigma: Notes on the Management of Spoiled Identity*. New Jersey: Prentice Hall Inc.

Goodwin, V.A. and Allan, L. (2019) 'Mrs Smith has no rehab potential': Does rehabilitation have a role in the management of people with dementia? *Age and Ageing*, 48, 1: 5–7.

Gove, D., Small, N., Downs, M. and Vernooij-Dassen, M. (2016) General practitioners' perceptions of the stigma of dementia and the role of reciprocity. *Dementia* (online publication) doi: 10.1177/1471301215625657 (accessed January 2018).

Hale, B., Barrett, P. and Gauld, R. (2010) *The Age of Supported Independence. Voice of In-home Care*. New York: Springer.

Harris, P.B. (2008) 'Another wrinkle in the debate about successful ageing': The undervalued concept of resilience and the lived experience of dementia. *International Journal of Aging and Human Development*, 67: 43–61.

Harrop, E., Addis, S., Elliot, E. and Williams, G. (2009) *Resilience, Coping and Salutogenic Approaches to Maintaining and Generating Health: A Review.* Cardiff: Cardiff Institute for Society, Health and Ethics.

Havighurst, R.J. (1961) Successful ageing. *The Gerontologist*, 1: 8–13.

Hedman, R., Hansebo, G., Ternestedt, B.M., Hellstrom, I. and Norberg, A. (2013) How people with Alzheimer's disease express their sense of self: Analysis using Rom Harré's theory of selfhood. *Dementia*, 12: 713–733.

Hicks, M.M. and Conner, N.E. (2014) Resilient ageing: A concept analysis. *Journal of Advanced Nursing*, 70 (4): 744–755.

Houston, A. and Christie, J. (2018) *Talking Sense: The Impact of Sensory Changes and Dementia.* Sydney: HammondCare.

Hughes, J.C., Louw, S.J. and Sabat, S.R. (2006) Seeing Whole. In: J.C. Hughes, S.J. Louw and S.R. Sabat (eds) *Dementia: Mind, Meaning and the Person.* Oxford: Oxford University Press.

Hulko, W. (2009) From 'not a big deal' to 'hellish': Experiences of older people with dementia. *Journal of Aging Studies*, 23: 131–144.

Jacobs, S., Xie, C., Reilly, S., Hughes, J. and Challis, D. (2009) Modernising social care services for older people: Scoping the United Kingdom evidence base. *Ageing and Society*, 29 (4): 497–538.

Jacobson, N. (1993) Experiencing recovery: A dimensional analysis of recovery narratives. *Psychiatric Rehabilitation Journal*, 23: 248–255.

Jalil, R., Huber, J.W., Sixsmith, S. and Dickens, G.L. (2017) Mental health nurses' emotions, exposure to patient aggression, attitudes to and use of coercive measures: Cross sectional questionnaire survey. *International Journal of Nursing Studies*, 75, 130–138.

Jaworska, A. (1997) Respecting the margins of agency: Alzheimer's patients and the capacity to value. *Philosophy and Public Affairs*, 28: 105–138.

Joint Improvement Team and NHS Health Scotland (2014) *Somewhere to go and something to do. Active and Healthy Ageing: An Action Plan for Scotland 2014–2016.* Edinburgh: JIT.

Johannessen, A. and Moller, A. (2013) Experiences of persons with early-onset dementia in everyday life: A qualitative study. *Dementia*, 12 (4): 410–424.

Keady, J., Williams, S. and Hughes-Roberts, J. (2007) 'Making mistakes': Using co-constructed inquiry to illuminate meaning and relationships in the early adjustment to Alzheimer's disease – a single case study approach. *Dementia*, 6 (3): 343–364.

Kelly, F. (2010) Abusive interaction: Research into locked wards for people with dementia. *Social Policy and Society*, 9 (2): 267–277.

Kelly, M.E. and O'Sullivan, M. (2015) *Strategies and Techniques for Cognitive Rehabilitation.* Dublin: The Alzheimer Society of Ireland, Trinity College Institute of Neuroscience.

Lifton, R.J. (1993) *The Protean Self: Human Resilience in an Age of Fragmentation.* New York: Basic Books.

Lindstrom, B. and Eriksson, M. (2006) Contextualising salutogenesis and Antonovsky in public health development. *Health Promotion International,* 21 (3): 238–244.

Luthar, S.S., Cicchetti, D. and Becker, B. (2000) The construct of resilience: A critical evaluation and guidelines for future work. *Child Development,* 71 (3): 543–562.

McCrae, R.R. and Costa Jr., P.T. (1997) Personal trait structure as a human universal. *American Psychologist,* 52 (5): 509.

McDonald, A., Dawson, C. and Heath, B. (2008) *The Impact of the Mental Capacity Act (2005) on Social Worker's Decision Making. A Report for SCIE.* Available at www.scie.org.uk/publications/mca/files/MCA_UEAImpactStudyJune2008.pdf (accessed January 2019).

Manthorpe, J. (2004) Risk Taking. In: A. Innes, C. Archibald and C. Murphy (eds) *Dementia and Social Inclusion: Marginalised Groups and Marginalised Areas of Dementia Research, Care and Practice.* London: Jessica Kingsley Publishers.

Marshall, M. (ed.) (2004) *Perspectives on Rehabilitation and Dementia.* London. Jessica Kingsley Publishers.

Masten, A., Best, K. and Garmezy, N. (1990) Resilience and development: Contributions from the study of children who overcome adversity. *Development and Psychopathology,* 2: 425–444.

Masten, A.S. (2001) Ordinary Magic: Resilience processes in development. *American Psychologist,* 56: 227–238.

Meléndez and Pitarque (2018) Wellbeing, resilience and coping: Are there differences between healthy older adults, adults with mild cognitive impairment, and adults with Alzheimer-type dementia? *Archives of Gerontology and Geriatrics,* 77: 38–43.

Mitchell, W. (2018) *Somebody I Used to Know.* London: Bloomsbury Publishing.

Nelis, S.M., Clare, L. and Whitaker, C.J. (2014) Attachment in people with dementia and their caregivers: A systematic review. *Dementia,* 13 (6): 747–767.

O'Connor, I., Hughes, M., Turney, D., Wilson, J. and Setterland, D. (2006) *Social Work and Social Care Practice.* London: Sage.

O'Connor C.M., Poulos C.J., Gresham, M. and Poulos, R.G. (2018) *Supporting Independence and Function in People Living with Dementia: A Technical Guide to the Evidence Supporting Re-Ablement Interventions.* Sydney: HammondCare Media.

Österholm, J.H. and Samuelsson. C. (2014) Orally positioning persons with dementia in assessment meetings. *Ageing and Society* (online publication) doi: 10.1017/So144686X13000755 (accessed January 2019).

Ottmann, G. and Maragoudaki, M. (2015) Fostering resilience in later life: A narrative approach involving people facing disabling circumstances, carers and members of minority groups. *Ageing and Society,* 35 (10): 2071–2099.

Pargament, K.I., Koenig, H.G. and Perez, L. (2000) The many methods of religious coping: Development and initial validation of the RCOPE. *Journal of Clinical Psychology,* 56 (4), 519–543.

Pearce, A., Clare, L. and Pistrang, N. (2002) Managing Sense of Self: Coping in the early stages of Alzheimer's disease, *Dementia*, 1 (2): 173–192.

Pool, J. (2018) *Reducing the Symptoms of Alzheimer's Disease and Other Dementias: A Guide to Personal Cognitive Rehabilitation Techniques*. London: Jessica Kingsley Publishers.

Prince, M., Prina, M. and Guerchet, M. (2013) *Alzheimer Disease International World Alzheimer Report 2013. Journey of Caring: An Analysis of Long-Term Care for Dementia*. London: ADI.

Radden, J. and Fordyce, J.M. (2006) Into the Darkness: Losing Identity with Dementia. In: J.C. Hughes, S.J. Louw and S.R. Sabat (eds) *Dementia: Mind, Meaning and the Person*. Oxford: Oxford University Press.

Rahman, S. (2018) *Living with Frailty: From Assets and Deficits to Resilience*. Abingdon, Oxon: Routledge.

Randall, W., Baldwin, C., McKenzie-Mohr, S., McKim, E. and Furlong, D. (2015) Narrative and resilience: A comparative analysis of how older adults story their lives. *Journal of Aging Studies*, 34: 155–161.

Reissman, C.K. (2008) *Narrative Methods for the Human Sciences*. London: Sage.

Ricoeur, P. (1992) *Oneself as Another* (trans. K. Blamey). Chicago: University of Chicago Press.

Robinson, E. (2002) Should People with Alzheimer's Disease Take Part in Research? In: H. Wilkinson (ed.) *The Perspectives of People with Dementia: Research Methods and Motivations*. London: Jessica Kingsley Publishers.

Robinson, L., Hutchings, D., Corner, L., Finch, T., Hughes, J., Brittain, K. and Bond, J. (2007) Balancing Rights and Risks: Conflicting perspectives in the management of wandering in dementia. *Health, Risk and Society*, 9 (4): 389–406.

Rowe, J.W and Khan, R.L. (1997) Successful aging. *Gerontologist*, 37 (4): 433–440.

Sabat, S.R. (2006) Mind, Meaning and Personhood in Dementia: The Effects of Positioning. In: J.C. Hughes, S.J. Louw and S.R. Sabat (eds) *Dementia: Mind, Meaning and the Person*. Oxford: Oxford University Press.

Scottish Dementia Working Group, Research Sub-Group (2014) Core principles for involving people with dementia in research: Innovative practice. *Dementia*, 13 (5): 680–685.

ScotCen Social Research and the Life Changes Trust (2015) *Attitudes to Dementia: Scottish Social Attitudes 2014*. Edinburgh: ScotCen Social Research.

ScotCen Social Research and the Life Changes Trust (2018) *Attitudes to Dementia: Scottish Social Attitudes 2017*. Edinburgh: ScotCen Social Research.

Sinnot, J.D. (2009) Complex thought and construction of the self in the face of old age and death. *Journal of Adult Development*, 16: 155–165.

Snowden, D. (1997) Ageing and Alzheimer's disease: Lessons from the nun study. *Gerontologist*, 37: 150–156.

Sorensen, L., Waldorff, F. and Waldemar, G. (2008) Coping with mild Alzheimer's disease. *Dementia*, 7 (3): 287–299.

Sova, R. and Sova. D.H. (2006) *Storyboards: A Dynamic Storytelling Tool. Presentation delivered to the Usability Professionals Association.* Available at http://teced.com/wp-content/uploads/2011/06/upa2006_storyboards_a_dynamic_storytelling_tool.pdf (accessed January 2019).

Stern, Y. (2012) Cognitive reserve in ageing and Alzheimer's disease. *The Lancet, Neurology. Personal View*, 11 (11): 1006–1012.

Stryker, S. (1968) Identity salience and role performance: The relevance of symbolic interaction theory for family research. *Journal of Marriage and Families*, 30: 558–564.

Swaffer, K. (2014) Dementia and Prescribed Dis-engagement.™ *Dementia*, 14 (1): 3–6.

Taylor, J.S. (2004) Salutogenesis as a framework for child protection: Literature review. *Journal of Advanced Nursing*, 45 (6): 633–643.

Taylor, B.B. (2018) 'Think You Right: I Am Not What I Am': Dialectical self-overcoming and the concept of resilience. *Spectra*, 6 (2): 20–36.

Tronto, J. (1994) *Moral Boundaries: A Political Argument for an Ethic of Care.* New York: Routledge.

UK Government (1998) *United Kingdom: Human Rights Act 1998. United Kingdom of Great Britain and Northern Ireland.* Available at www.legislation.gov.uk/ukpga/1998/42/contents (accessed February 2019).

UK Government (2010) *Equality Act 2010. United Kingdom of Great Britain and Northern Ireland.* Available at www.legislation.gov.uk/ukpga/2010/15/contents (accessed February 2019).

United Nations (1948) *The Universal Declaration of Human Rights.* Available at www.ohchr.org/EN/UDHR/Documents/UDHR_Translations/eng.pdf (accessed February 2019).

United Nations (2006) *United Nations Convention on the Rights of the Person with Disabilities.* Available at https://www.un.org/disabilities/documents/convention/convention_accessible_pdf.pdf (accessed October 2019).

Walker, A. (2006) Active ageing in employment: Its meaning and potential. *Asia-Pacific Review*, 13: 78–95.

Wilson, G. and Fearnley, K. (2007) *The Dementia Epidemic: Where Scotland is Now and the Challenge Ahead.* Edinburgh: Alzheimer Scotland.

Windle, G. (2011) What is resilience? A review and concept analysis. *Reviews in Clinical Gerontology*, 21 (2): 152–169.

Windle, G. (2015) *Psychological Resilience: An Important Resource in Later Life?* In: The 2015 International Psychogeriatrics Association Annual Conference, Berlin, 13–16 October 2015.

Wolfe, A. (1997) Public and Private in Theory and Practice: Some Implications of an Uncertain Boundary. In: J. Weintraub and K. Kumar (eds) *Public and Private in Thought and Practice: Perspectives on a Grand Dichotomy.* Chicago: University of Chicago.

World Health Organization (2012) *Dementia: A Public Health Priority.* Geneva: WHO.

World Health Organization (2015a) *World Report on Ageing and Health.* Luxembourg: WHO.

World Health Organization (2015b) Ensuring a Human Rights Based Approach for People Living with Dementia. *Thematic Briefing.* WHO.

World Health Organization (2017) *Strengthening Resilience: A Priority Shared by Health 2020 and the Sustainable Development Goals.* Denmark: WHO.

Young, E. (2010) Narrative therapy and elders with memory loss. *Clinical Social Work Journal,* 38: 193–202.

Young, J.A, Lind, C., Orange, J.B. and Savundranayagam, M.Y. (2019) Expanding current understandings of epistemic injustice and dementia: Learning from stigma theory. *Journal of Aging Studies,* 48: 76–84.

Zeisel, J., Reisberg, B., Whitehouse, P., Woods, R. and Verheul, A. (2016) Ecopsychosocial interventions in cognitive decline and dementia: A new terminology and a new paradigm. *American Journal of Alzheimer's Disease and Other Dementias,* 31 (6): 502–507.

Subject Index

acceptance, re-framing 137–40
adaptive capacity 42
adjustment
  dealing with loss 92
  personal theories as
    essential part of 101
  re-framing resignation and
    acceptance as 137–40
  as stage of self-maintenance 39
Adult Support and Protection
  (Scotland) Act (2007) 54
adversity
  buffers in face of 20, 79–80, 83–5
  discussing experiences of 130
  experience of dementia as 105
  of human service
    practitioners 163
  reflections on 94–7
  resilience developed in
    face of 19, 23–4, 105
ageing
  attitudes to 36–8, 64, 79
  healthy 32
  as life adversity 62
  personal theories about 98–101
  policy context 32–3
  as strength in development
    of resilience 78
  successful 35
ageism 26, 37
Alan 52–3, 68–70, 74, 86–7,
  90–1, 96–7, 138

assessment
  approaching from narrative or
    storytelling perspective 107–9
  location of 111–12
  planning for 110–11
  purpose of 106
  reflecting position, values and
    focus of practitioner 106–7
  types of 128–9
  used to engage 135–6
assessment process 106,
  110–12, 114, 162
asset-based approaches 55–9
asset mapping 55–6
assets
  of Jakub 144
  of Jane 147
  mobilisation and employment
    of 105, 115
  as resilience domain 118
  types 55, 107
  valuable repository of 166–7
  visualising 55–6, 105–6
attachment theory 85–6
autobiographical reasoning
  78–9, 95–6
autonomy 33, 128, 136–7

Beth 50–1, 93–4, 100–1, 129–30
brain 12, 45–6
buffers in face of adversity
  20, 79–80, 83–5

care ethics 53–4
Charles 139–40
citizenship
    as active process 65
    aspects of dementia 58
    assessments revealing 108
    failure to recognise status of 139
    losing domestic 62, 138
    models of dementia 54
    narrative 78
    new model of 166
    practice focused on 116
    resilience concerned with 27, 54
    rights 137
    taking many forms 27–8
cognitive reserve 45–50
Colin 153–5
compensation strategies 46
connectedness
    association with attachment
      theory 85
    in dementia resilience matrix 85
    examples in action 85–8
    of Jakub 144–5
    of Jane 148
    of Noreen 119–20
    as protective factor 20–1, 83–4
    in quick rating tool 102
    risk factors 88
    of William 150
control see mastery and control
co-production 57–9, 124–5

dementia
    and assessment 106–7, 110–11
    and attachment 86–8
    co-production 58–9
    dealing with forgetfulness 123
    denial of impact example 153–5
    everyday stories of life with
      importance of 107–10
      as rich repositories of
        information 113–14, 166–7
      setting scene 111–12
    expectations of others 137–40
    expressions of threats to
      sense of self 67–71
    as global health priority 34
    hearing people with 78
    and identity 63–6
    independence 136, 141
    interdependence 53–5
    intersecting experiences
      52–3, 130
    as life adversity 62
    'living well' with 34–5
    mastery and control 89–90, 156
    matrices
      experience 81
      resilience 85
    meaning making 94–101
    and motivation 50–1
    nature of 24
    organisational processes and
      priorities 128–9, 141
    personal theories about 98–101
    person with versus people
      with 133–6, 155
    and policy 34–6
    positioning 92–3
    protective factors 20, 83
    reserve capacity and cognitive
      reserve 45–6, 48–50
    and resilience
      and ageing 38
      applicability 25–6
      benefits 166–7
      discourse 165–6
      experience 38–40, 105
      framework for support
        115–16, 166
      and human rights 41–2
      learning from 160–1
      opportunity 27–8
      possibility 61–3, 127, 160
      potential and realisation 35–6
      realising 160–1
      thinking differently about 59–60
      as window into life 161–2
    and risk
      accepting limits 141
      focus on 127
      living with 131–2
    salutogenesis 57

and social competence 89
and survival 73–6
thinking differently about
    45, 59–60, 73, 156
dementia network,
    resilience of 163–5
dementia resilience matrix 85
dependent independence 136–7
'doing okay' 39, 87, 97–8,
    101, 144, 147
Dora 67–8, 70, 91–2, 98–9
Doug 134, 138–9

economy 63
eco-psycho-social approach 27
Ellen 36–7, 70, 95, 97
epistemic injustice 69–70, 133
Equality Act (2010) 41
European Convention on
    Human Rights (ECHR) 41
everyday magic 109–10
everyday, prioritising 123–4
expectations of others 137–40
experiences
    of ageing 64
    of Beth 130–1
    dementia as not eroding 166
    of Jakub 145
    of Jane 148
    motivations shaped by 51
    of Noreen 121–2
    relation to meaning making 84
    as resilience domain 117
    in Resilience Reserve 47, 115
    totality of 52
    use of previous 97
    value of 27–8, 166–7

Fathimaa 146–52
frailty 33, 38, 134
functional ability 32–3

good enough
    developing own measure of 97–8
    externally imposed views of 25
Gwen 128–9, 138

healthy ageing 32
Helen 93–4, 129–30, 134–6
human rights 27–8, 41–2, 54, 88
Human Rights Act (1998) 41, 54
'hyper presence' 76

Ian 139–40
identity
    everyday activities as
        foundations of 159
    expressions of 67–71
    impact of 'frail' 33
    life cycle stages 63–4
    organisational 127–31
    person with dementia 132
    and positioning 89–90, 92
    resilience important for
        preservation of 166
    as shaped by telling
        stories 76, 84, 160
    spoiled 66–7
    survivor 75
    symbolic interactionist
        perspectives 64–6
    see also sense of self
'identity continuum' 66
ill-being 55, 88
independence
    as catalyst for resilience
        process 42–3
    central role of 141
    definition 136
    dementia seen as affecting 49
    dependent 136–7
    as indicator of successful
        ageing 35
    relation with resilience 25–6, 34
    risks versus 54
    supported 136
injustices 69–70
interdependence 53–5
intersectionality 51–3, 152

Jakub 143–5
Jane 146–9, 151–2
John 61–2

Kate 136–7
knowledge, skills and interests
    Jakub 144
    Jane 147
    as mastery and control
        factor 21, 84
    Noreen 121–2
    as resilience domain 117
    in Resilience Reserve 47

Lottie 152–3

magic
    everyday 109–10
    'magical thinking' 70
    'ordinary' 109, 160
Mary 143–5
mastery and control
    in dementia resilience matrix 85
    examples in action 88–94
    experiencing loss of 57
    explanation 21, 84
    Jane 149
    Noreen 120
    as protective factor 20, 83
    in quick rating tool 102
    and support 140
    William 150
Maura 155–6
meaning making
    in dementia resilience matrix 85
    examples in action 94–101
    explanation 21, 84
    Jane 149
    Noreen 120
    as protective factor 20, 83
    in quick rating tool 102
    William 151
Michael 119–23
motivation
    Jakub 144
    Jane 147
    new concept of 50–1
    Noreen 121
    as resilience domain 119
    in Resilience Reserve 47

narrative assessment process 110–11
narrative openness 78–9, 91, 95
narrative self 76–9
'neoliberal subjects' 34
Noreen 119–23
'Nun Study' 46

opportunity, resilience as 27–8
organisational identity 127–31

PANEL principles 42
Paul 155–6
personal accountability 33–4
personal qualities
    Jakub 145
    Jane 148
    as resilience domain 118
    in Resilience Reserve 47
'person in situation' 124–5
policy
    and dementia 34–6
    and resilience 32–4
positioning
    explanation 89–90
    malignant social example 69
    re-positioning within
        stories 90–4, 114, 162
    social competence linked to 89
practice scenarios
    Colin 153–5
    Jakub 143–5
    Jane and William 146–52
    Maura 155–6
    Sunil and Lottie 152–3
practice tensions
    competing demands 128–31
    dependent independence 136–7
    expectations of others 137–40
    living with risk 131–6
    overview 127, 140–1
'prescribed disengagement' 93
protective factors
    acting as buffers in face of
        adversity 20, 79–80, 83–5
    connectedness 85–8
    Fathimaa
        for Jane 148–9
        for William 150–1

Lottie 152–3
mastery and control 88–94
Maura 156
meaning making 94–102
Michael 120–1
promoting through targeted
    resources 19
quick rating tool 101–3
relation with risk 81, 87–8
relation with vulnerability 80–1
and resilience 144–5, 146–9, 156
three main 20, 83

re-ablement 48–50, 136, 160
rehabilitation 48–50, 136, 160
religious coping 99
reserve capacity 45–50
resignation, re-framing 137–40
resilience
    and ageing 36–8
    brief history 31–2
    definition 19
    and dementia
        and ageing 38
        applicability 25–6
        benefits 166–7
        discourse 165–6
        experience 38–40, 105
        framework for support
            115–16, 166
        and human rights 41–2
        learning from 160–1
        possibility 61–3, 127, 160
        potential and realisation 35–6
        realising 160–1
        thinking differently about 59–60
        as window into life 161–2
    of dementia network 163–5
    factors acting as catalysts for 42–3
    nature of 23–4, 59
    as opportunity 27–8
    policy context 32–4
    practice tensions in
        search for 127–40
    problem with 26
    and protective factors
        144–5, 146–9, 156

realising
    with dementia 160–1
    four steps 19–20
    practice scenarios 143–57
    supporting 35–6
resilience discourse 165–6
resilience domains 117–18
resilience-focused example 119–23
resilience matrix 84–5
resilience model 19–21, 166
Resilience Reserve 19–21,
    46–50, 115–23, 164
resources
    accumulation of 19, 33
    asset-based approaches 55–9
    best utilisation of 105–6, 166–7
    in dementia resilience matrix 85
    external 32, 49
    flexible cognitive 46
    Jakub 144
    Jane 147–8
    lack of, as source of stress 38
    Lottie 152
    organisational gatekeeping
        to access 128
    people with fewest 60
    pooled 116, 163
    in realising resilience 19–20
    as resilience domain 118
    in Resilience Reserve
        46–7, 101–2, 164
    state role in provision of 34
risk
    close association with
        dementia 127, 141
    facilitating resilience
        by reducing 19
    focus on 26, 127
    independence versus 54
    living with 131–6
    of losing self 160
    of low self-esteem 93
    negative impact 20
    over-emphasis on 25, 41
    vulnerability and protective
        factors 79–81
risk continuum 81, 85

risk factors
  Jane 148–9
  Lottie 152–3
  Noreen 119–21
  quick rating tool 101–2
  thematic relationship with
    protective factors 87–8
  William 150–1
roles
  Charles 139–40
  Jakub 145
  Jane 148
  Noreen 121
  of practitioners 132, 141
  as resilience domain 117
  in Resilience Reserve 47
  support resulting in loss of 140

salutogenesis 56–7
self
  continuation of 97–8, 131
  holding on to
    despite changing
      circumstances 160
    preservation of 66
    through narrative and story 76
  loss of 66, 81, 160
  presentations in social
    interaction 64–6
  re-positioning within
    stories 90–4, 114, 162
  see also narrative self; sense of self
self-confidence 115
self-efficacy 85, 88, 93,
  102, 120, 149–50
self-esteem 55, 85, 88–9, 93,
  102, 120, 149–50
self-image 33, 59, 82
self-maintenance 39
self-recognition 159
self-reflection 64
self-stigma 88
'sense of coherence' 56
sense of self
  in experience of dementia
    matrix 81
  expressions of threats to 67–71

holding on to 73–82
importance of
  connectedness 20–1
  memory loss having profound
    impact on 123
  organisational identity
    versus 128–31
  power of stories 82, 101, 108
  in resilience definition 19
  see also identity
social competence 89
spoiled identity 66–7
stigma 26, 33, 62–3, 88, 93–4
stories
  benefits 161–2
  as demonstrations of
    resilience in action 165
  learning from 109–10
  of life with dementia
    call to create better 167
    importance of 107–10
  narrative self 76–9
  'person in situation' 124–5
  recognising reflections of
    identity in 160–1
  re-positioning self within
    90–4, 114, 162
  rich with expressions
    of identity 71
  scene-setting 111–12
storyboards 112–14, 162
'successful ageing' 35
Sunil 152–3
'supported independence' 136
survival 73–6, 97
symbolic interactionist
  perspectives 64–6

Tanya 153–5
therapeutic nihilism 48–9
threats
  emotional 62
  to identity
    in resilience definition 19
    use of positioning 92–3
  to sense of self, expressions
    of 67–71

UN Convention on Rights of
  Persons with Disabilities 41
Universal Declaration of
  Human Rights 41

vulnerability 25, 79–81
vulnerability factors 39, 80,
  83, 109, 161, 166
vulnerable 34, 80, 89–90, 129

wellbeing
  absence of ill-health not
    necessarily equating to 56–7
  as aspiration causing
    undue pressure 35
  of carers 28, 115–16, 163–4
  connectedness for 20, 84
  everyday activities promoting 48
  focus on health 98
  impact of spoiled identity 66
  indicator of, for Ellen 95
  relationships with negative
    impact on 86, 88
  and resilience 23, 62, 132
  suffering with dementia
    indicating absence of 75
  and vulnerable 80
Wendy 77
William 146–7, 150–2

Author Index

Abbema, R.V. 38
Allan, L. 48
Allen, R.S. 79
Alzheimer Disease International 34
Antonovsky, A. 56
Auburn, T. 65

Bailey, C. 40, 131–2
Baldwin, C. 78
Barnes, M. 137
Barnes, R. 65
Barrett, P. 136
Barry, M. 131, 134
Bartlett, R. 27, 62, 69
Batsch, N. 63
Bavidge, M. 35, 38
Becker, B. 23
Bennett, K.M. 38
Berger, P.L. 90
Best, K. 31
Bowes, A. 38
Bowlby, J. 85
Bowling, A. 35
Brannelly, T. 137
Bubeck, D. 53
Butler, R.N. 35, 37, 64

Caddell, L. 63–4
Cations, M. 49
Chandler, D. 34
Charon, J.M. 65

Christie, J. 49, 111
Cicchetti, D. 23
Clare, L. 39, 48, 63–4, 86, 160
Clarke, C.L. 40, 131–2
Clark, P.G. 38
Conner, N.E. 35, 56
Costa, P.T., Jr. 64
Coulshed, V. 124
Cox, S. 111
Crenshaw-Williams, K. 51
Cuddy, A.J. 38

Daniel, B. 16, 38, 47, 85
Dawson, C. 132
De Beauvoir, S. 63
Department of Health 63
Dias, R. 38
Dieppe, P. 35

Erikson, E.H. 63–4
Eriksson, M. 56
European Court of Human Rights 41

Fearnley, K. 63
Fiske, S.T. 38
Fordyce, J.M. 75–6
Forstmeier, S. 51, 160
Fricker, M. 69
Friedland, R. 56–7

Garmezy, N. 31
Gauld, R. 136
Giebel, C.M. 48
Goffman, E. 64–7
Goodwin, V.A. 48
Gove, D. 63
Guerchet, M. 63

Hale, B. 136
Harris, P.B. 39, 87, 97
Harrop, E. 56–7
Havighurst, R.J. 35
Heath, B. 132
Hedman, R. 86
Hicks, M.M. 35, 56
Houston, A. 49, 111
Hughes, J.C. 63, 160
Hughes-Roberts, J. 39
Hulko, W. 52, 57, 100, 130, 160

Jacobson, N. 99
Jacobs, S. 16
Jalil, R. 164
Jaworska, A. 75
Johannessen, A. 69
Joint Improvement Team 63

Kahn, R.L. 35
Keady, J. 39
Kelly, F. 90
Kelly, M.E. 49
Koenig, H.G. 99

Lea, S. 65
Lifton, R.J. 73
Lindstrom, B. 56
Louw, S.J. 63, 160
Luckman, T. 90
Luthar, S.S. 23

Maercker, A. 51, 160
Manthorpe, J. 132
Maragoudaki, M. 51
Marshall, M. 48
Masten, A.S. 23, 31, 160
McCrae, R.R. 64

McDonald, A. 132
Meléndez, J.C. 70
Mitchell, W. 76–7
Mittelman, S. 63
Moller, A. 69

Nelis, S.M. 86
NHS Health Scotland 63
Norton, M.I. 38

O'Connor, C.M. 49
O'Connor, D. 27
O'Connor, I. 106
Orme, J. 124
Österholm, J.H. 106–7, 138
O'Sullivan, M. 49
Ottmann, G. 51

Pargament, K.I. 99
Pearce, A. 39
Perez, L. 99
Pistrang, N. 39
Pitarque, A. 70
Pool, J. 49
Prina, M. 63
Prince, M. 63

Radden, J. 75–6
Rahman, S. 33
Randall, W. 79, 91
Reid, J. 34
Reissman, C.K. 76
Ricoeur, P. 68, 74
Robinson, E. 112
Robinson, L. 131
Rowe, J.W. 35

Sabat, S.R. 63, 69, 90, 93, 160, 162
Samuelsson. C. 106–7, 138
ScotCen Social Research and
    the Life Changes Trust 62
Scottish Dementia Working Group,
    Research Sub-Group 111
Shakespeare, P. 39
Sinnot, J.D. 37
Snowden, D. 46

Sorensen, L. 69
Sova, D.H. 112
Sova, R. 112
Stern, Y. 46
Stryker, S. 65
Sutcliffe, C. 48
Swaffer, K. 93

Taylor, B.B. 68
Taylor, J.S. 57
Tronto, J. 53

UK Government 41, 54
United Nations (UN) 41

Waldemar, G. 69
Waldorff, F. 69
Walker, A. 35
Wassell, S. 16, 47, 85
Whitaker, C.J. 86
Williams, S. 39
Wilson, G. 63
Windle, G. 38, 57
Wolfe, A. 64
World Health Organization
    32, 41–2, 63

Young, E. 108, 162
Young, J.A. 70, 133

Zeisel, J. 27